EPILEPSY UNVEILED

EPILEPSY UNVEILED

Caretaking, Seizures, Psychosis and Brain Surgery

Lola Jines-Burritt

www.epilepsyunveiled.com

ISBN 978-0-9852402-0-2
Library of Congress Catalog Control Number: 2012904066
Epilepsy Unveiled: Caretaking, Seizures, Psychosis and Brain Surgery/ by Lola Jines-Burritt

Note: This publication contains the opinions and ideas of its author. It is intended to provide helpful and informative material on the subject matter covered. It is sold with the understanding that the author and publisher are not engaged in rendering professional or medical services. If the reader requires personal assistance or medical advice a competent medical professional should be consulted.

The author and publisher specifically disclaim any responsibility for any liability, loss, or risk, personal or otherwise, which is incurred as a consequence, directly or indirectly of the use and application of any contents of this book.

Contents

I dedicate this book to my loving husband Bobby whose unconditional love and encouragement has helped bring my book to life. I am sure it is not easy sharing your present life with my past one, but you never complain. Bobby, your kind heart has taught me how to live again. I love you more every day.

I thank Dr. Bruce Mickey for taking the time to read the first (very) rough draft of this book and teaching me through words of wisdom and encouragement how to make improvements. Being advised by a famous brain surgeon is an honor I do not take lightly.

Introduction

The one perfectly clear fact regarding epilepsy is the questions are endless and answers few. Unanswered questions lead to living in isolation surrounded by walls that are constructed by piling up fear, confusion, misunderstanding, social stigmas and the mistake of hiding behaviors that are the creation of multiple seizures. These pages contain details of the journey my husband, Charley, and I traveled as we dealt with his epilepsy while living behind closed doors for twenty-six years.

Life with epilepsy can be compared to a puzzle. The picture on the front of the puzzle box is beautiful. Inside the box are jumbled pieces that no one can take out and instantly find a match for. This book takes pieces of the puzzle epilepsy created for Charley and I and puts them together to help create a frame of comprehension for people who are now living with seizures. Life with epilepsy, as you know, needs to be more understandable.

This book is for those who feel blindfolded as they journey down the unfamiliar paths epilepsy creates. Each chapter contains information that represents a new door opened by the hands of strength and perseverance. When dealing with epilepsy strength does count and determination can defeat seizures.

If you are living behind closed doors because of epilepsy step out of isolation and find new ways to cope. Use the answers provided that apply to your life and build a frame of comprehension for your puzzle pieces. Never allow epilepsy to take the beauty out of the picture that is the creation of your life.

Epilepsy Unveiled

Preface

Charley and I met in 1980 working at a construction job. He was a carpenter and I a young woman working as a carpenter's helper; a field I knew nothing about. Charley became my protector and shared his carpentry knowledge. We became friends as he patiently taught me how to lay out and frame walls. Charley's every stride spoke confidence. He had beautiful blue eyes, wavy brownish hair and a red goatee. I later found out when his goatee was pulled it caused him to baa like a goat. He was a rough looking man who had been in many fights resulting in a crooked nose. Children were intimidated by Charley's looks but he could usually persuade them to pull his beard resulting in a long baa that instantly transformed an intimidating looking man into a fun friend.

I was a single mother when I met Charley. At twenty three years old I was prettier than I knew and dumber than I thought. Looking back it is clear at that time in my life I needed to be needed. Eventually Charley and I began dating and when his first seizure occurred I was drawn in like a moth to a flame. Charley was a hard working man whose life would have been very monetarily successful, I am sure, had it not been for epilepsy. In spite of seizures we managed to live a successful life and adored each other for many reasons; a glue that held our marriage together for twenty-six years.

Prior to our marriage Charley had a few seizures, but we were not overly-concerned. For several years his seizures were controlled by medication but as time passed more seizures occurred. When Charley was diagnosed with temporal lobe epilepsy (his seizures originated in his left temporal lobe) we dealt with the harsh reality that life was not going to be easy and carried on with our journeys through a team effort. Charley suffered with every imaginable type of seizure and his condition progressively worsened. We coped with seizures and erratic behavior for more than twenty years before he was diagnosed with clusters of seizures that were causing postictal psychosis.

On one occasion I felt cheated by the burdens imposed upon me and was heartsick over the troubles epilepsy created. As I cursed our circumstances and selfishly prayed for relief the Lord whispered a message to my soul saying, "Charley is your lesson in life, stop trying to change him and be observant." I knew we were together for a reason, but I falsely assumed that was because Charley needed me. As time passed I grudgingly applied the Lord's message and slowly comprehended the mental and physical toll Charley paid because of epilepsy. My burdens were light compared to his. Putting aside my self-importance helped me discover, and cherish, how much I loved my husband. I became stronger throughout the years and Charley inevitably became weaker because of the growing severity of his seizures. While he miserably lived epilepsy from the inside out our roles reversed and I became his protector as I lived epilepsy from the outside in.

In 2002 Charley became debilitated by clusters of seizures. He had several seizures a day and was chronically psychotic. Faced with the choice of having constant seizures and the fear of entirely losing his sanity, he chose to have his left temporal lobe removed. Charley had no more seizures or behaviors caused by postictal psychosis after surgery. As he healed life settled down, and for the first time in our marriage we were no longer ruled by seizures. However; the conditioning seizures had instilled in our life tormented us both. We were not prepared for this journey but stubbornly continued on thinking somewhere ahead there had to be a light at the end of the tunnel.

I began writing this book in 2003, shortly before Charley's brain surgery. The experience has been incredible. Writing became my best friend as I took care of Charley when seizures incapacitated him. I scratched words on the pages of a spiral notebook outside a surgery unit in Dallas, Texas while my husband's left temporal lobe was being removed by a team of surgeons. I watched over Charley as he healed and continued recording our experiences while I made sure he was comfortable, nourished and bathed. I pecked away at my keyboard and left him alone when he began a seizure-free life so he could keep his thoughts gathered and complete tasks he was trying to accomplish. Writing was my occupation as I learned how not to follow Charley everywhere waiting to catch him as I constantly watched for a seizure to occur.

I stopped writing in 2005 because Charley became very sick. He was diagnosed with hepatitis c. He had taken medications for many years and his liver was failing. I realized our journeys, after nearly twenty-six years, were concluding. We spent every moment together and on August 16th of 2006, Charley died of liver failure. It took a while to start writing again after his death but I forced myself to continue, thinking I only lacked a few months and this book would be finished. It has now been nine years since I began writing. I want every seizure Charley endured to count toward helping others.

I have several goals for this book. The first is to pass on my knowledge, give concrete advice and offer suggestions that will advance everyone who is trying to cope with epilepsy beyond the unknown. I hope to create a better understanding for families who are experiencing epilepsy from the outside in and the true victims of seizures who are living with epilepsy from the inside out.

Another goal is to speak to people who have epilepsy and suffer with clusters of seizures and postictal psychosis. Our experiences can help them understand their illness so they no longer feel lost and alone. Psychotic behavior is not normal, but according to medical experts who specialize in the field of epilepsy postictal psychosis caused by clusters of seizures is known to occur in six to ten percent of people who have epilepsy. That is a lot of people.

I want to prevent individuals and their families (who are considering brain surgery) from falling off of some of the emotional cliffs we plummeted down after Charley's surgery. Unexpected changes will occur when seizures are eliminated. Everyone's experiences after brain surgery will be different but I guarantee there will be struggles.

Helping others build strength as they travel down the many roads living with epilepsy creates is another of my goals. Most of my strength was built through prayer and observance. Learning to suck in my breath as I spoke to myself and then praying rather than speaking so I could observe Charley (rather than correct him) helped me understand and cope. Each chapter in this book represents a piece of our life that I survived because of the strength my prayers instilled within my heart and the answers those prayers brought to my mind during my darkest moments. I am far from a saint. There were many times as tears rolled down my face that I prayed and cursed our circumstances within the same breath. None of the roads we traveled were easy but we proceeded with our journeys the best we could. I hope you benefit from traveling with us.

Charley's Poem

Love of my life
Please Comprehend
This is the beginning
Not the end
Life is only what we make it
Not what has been.

I try every day to please you
Although I'm coming across
Different than I project.
I know that you love me.
I hope you can deflect
This feeling of rejection.

I love you more than life itself.
Please accept me
And all my flaws
As many as there are,
Not loving you
Is not one of them.

Written by Charley Ross Jines to Lola Jines –1991

Living
with
Epilepsy

Epilepsy Unveiled

Chapter 1

Those Pesky Seizures: Endure and Learn

As the partner or caretaker of a person who has seizures you will go through a long period of adjustment as you learn to deal with the new world seizures produce. The person you take care of is not aware of the true circumstances that seizures create. They are not conscious while you brace them or keep them from falling. Your soul listens and tunes into them as their system is tuning out everything due to a seizure.

You cannot guess when a seizure will occur but eventually you will learn how to always be prepared, brace for seizures, and listen for seizure indicators. At first you will doubt your inner warning system. For a while, though some little voice told you the person you love is going to have a seizure, you will watch them fall before you learn to trust the fact that a warning alarm has developed within you that sounds seconds before a seizure occurs. When you recognize that you are an insider, one of the few people who really understands and tunes into seizures, you will observe and try to stay one step ahead of the person who has seizures. You will always be alert as you watch and listen for something the person you love is not aware of and has never witnessed. Trust your instincts, they grow slowly as far as seizures are concerned but those instincts are tried and true.

The person who has seizures is aware of your actions when they are not having a seizure but they have moaned or made a noise that triggers your seizure alert system. When they have triggered your alert system and you run toward them like a possessed idiot and grab them like superman to brace them for a fall they may think you have lost your mind. When Charley startled me with anything my system thought was a seizure alert he used to say, "Lo, what the hell are you doing?" as I grabbed him and braced both of us for a fall. His exasperated exclamation was a relief. Unsound the alarm. No seizure this time. Yahoo!!

There are many different types of seizures but they are not the only physically obvious result of owning a brain that misfires. Falling down and convulsing are only a few of the unpredictable behaviors inaccurate brain signals cause. Charley did not always have seizures when his brain misfired. Often his crossed signals created milder behaviors such as muscle spasms, twitches, severe itching, neck aches, mispronounced words, inappropriate verbalization, drooling, finger tapping, repeatedly gagging, and being suddenly disoriented.

I often wondered how many misfires he had that I could not see compared to the times I witnessed a vague, clumsy movement or saw the physical results of his inaccurate brain signals. I bet for every one "misfiring neuron" behavior I witnessed there were probably a thousand incidences Charley endured but could not describe, and did not know how they influenced his everyday behaviors.

Be prepared for all circumstances seizures create. Sometimes you will see seizures if you are with someone whose brain misfires and others you will see that person's body or mind in misery as the result of misfiring neurons, but there will be no seizure. For Charley and I the visible seizures were the beginning of epilepsy. Seeing someone have seizures makes epilepsy very real. As you tune into the person who has seizures watch for pre-seizure behaviors. Be aware of actions they display at the initial onset of a seizure such as teeth grinding, moaning, tremors, crying or lashing out in anger. Pre-seizure behaviors are your warning to instantly prepare yourself to catch, brace, or comfort the person in case they do have a seizure.

Something always happens within the brain before a seizure occurs. One of our greatest struggles was realizing the physical reactions Charley's body displayed because of seizures were only a small part of the overall picture of epilepsy.

You will eventually learn not to feel too stupid about trying to catch a person when they are not having a seizure but you will never be able to shake off the guilt when that person falls and hurts themselves, whether you are with them or they are alone. Seizure instincts create a protective and caring person that cannot tolerate seeing the physical bumps and bruises on the person they love that are caused by seizures. I could not always protect Charley from the hazards of seizures but I did my best as I am sure you will. Following are a few tips about seizure types and caretaking.

When a **tonic-clonic** (when Charley started having seizures these were called grand-mal, their new medical name is tonic-clonic), atonic seizure (drop attack), or myoclonic (jerks) that cause someone to fall occurs and there is time at the onset of the seizure stand behind them and tuck your arms under their arms and tightly around the front of their chest. Glue your body to theirs with your knees against the back of their knees (or legs) and slightly pull them toward you while firmly pulling them against your chest. As your arms balance the top of their body hold your back straight and slowly push your knees forward against the back of their knees (or legs, the point is to get their knees to bend). Their legs will be stiff. Pushing against their knees puts you in control of their knees bending forward and the beginning of the fall that both of you are going to take. Go down to the floor with them as you hold them firmly against you and take control of their body. Don't try to hold them up (that is not going to happen) or attempt to keep them from falling if you are unable to. When a body plummets downward it is impossible to stop. Be prepared to cushion the fall with control and not force. **(Only do this if you have the strength to control their fall and you are healthy enough withstand being their cushion).** After the person is lying down, and you have managed to untangle yourself, turn them on their side to protect their airway, loosen their clothes and let the seizure pass as you speak comforting words. Charley never knew how many times he nearly squished the life out of me because I absorbed the brunt of his falls but he felt my presence and knew I was taking care of him.

Charley began tonic-clonic seizures with a loud, eerily disturbing moan and his arms went straight out from his body (which scared the dickens out of more than one stranger). He was extremely stiff as he, or we, fell to the floor followed by jerking, slobbering and loss of bladder control.

Another problem is created by the loss of bladder control. At home I used a hand-held urinal to catch Charley's urine. Sometimes I could not get him in a position to use a urinal so I poked an adult diaper or a towel around the areas I expected to get wet and hoped for the best.

Have an adult diaper handy and keep a waterproof mattress pad on the bed. If urine leaks onto the mattress mix a teaspoon of bleach with water in a thirty-two ounce spray bottle and spray that on the wet area of the mattress. Then put on rubber gloves and spread a thick layer of baking soda on top of the wet spot. Mash the soda into the mattress with your hands and keep putting it on the wet spot until the lower layer is a paste and the top layer a bit dry. Turn a fan on low and place it beside the spot so it will blow onto the paste of baking soda and keep the fan running until the baking soda and mattress are dry. After the baking soda completely dries vacuum it and the mattress is fine.

Loss of bladder control in public because of a seizure is a nuisance but do not let that be an embarrassment. Most strangers witnessing a seizure are quite shaken and have no idea loss of bladder control happened. So . . . act like it did not happen. After Charley's unexpected seizures I sat on the floor in many public places with his head on my lap and body sprawled out beside me. We have been completely surrounded by puzzled people as I nonchalantly waited for him to recover enough to get up and walk. Total strangers have helped me get Charley off of the floor and a few have helped me load him onto a flat cart or wheelchair and roll him to our vehicle. I honestly do not think they noticed Charley's loss of bladder control. If they did nothing was said. Do not make a big issue out of the loss of bladder control.

Few elements of living with epilepsy are black and white but occasional loss of bladder control is. A person with epilepsy lives an ever-changing, unpredictable life. When seizures create gray areas they have to be confronted on an individual basis. If seizures increase in frequency or intensity the gray areas change. Patiently observe the person who has seizures and apply a process of trial and error to discover and make familiar the unknowns that exist in the gray areas of your life. Constantly expand your gray area knowledge and apply that knowledge to make your life as enjoyable as possible.

When the person you love has a seizure do your best to protect them from injury. Cushion their head and calmly reassure them. Do not restrain them, put anything in their mouth, or move them. One mistake I made when Charley had seizures took a while to comprehend. The day after having had seizures his throat was raw and he had a bad lingering taste in his mouth. He hated going to the hospital so between seizures occurring I gave him oral medication. Charley was barely lucid when I woke him, poked medicine in his mouth and made him drink water. I did not pay attention to how much water Charley drank. We eventually realized I was not making him drink enough water when he swallowed the medication. The pills were sticking in his throat and dissolving; therefore making it raw. If giving oral medication to a person after a seizure make them sit up and drink enough water to completely wash the pills down.

Absence or Petit Mal seizures are said to be more common in children and teenagers but Charley constantly had them. He appeared to be daydreaming but was actually momentarily unconscious and totally unaware of what was happening around him, even though his eyes were open. When a person has these seizures it looks like they are staring but the gaze lasts too long. If the person who has epilepsy realizes they have missed a few minutes because of the seizure fill in the blank. I usually ignored Charley's staring and did not tell him what he missed. He did not realize time had passed while he was unaware of his surroundings and my filling him in confused him more than the seizure. Do not shake the person with epilepsy or shout at them if they are staring. At times I gently nudged Charley which helped bring him out of an absence seizure.

Absence seizures occur more often in unfamiliar environments. I always dreaded Charley having absence seizures in public. He usually felt something was amiss if he came out of a seizure and perfect strangers were staring at him. He had no clue that he had blanked out.

Many years ago Charley, our daughter Kate, and I were in a group counseling session with several other families. Each parent introduced themselves and their child. When it was Charley's turn he was staring. Katie and I knew he was having a mild seizure. I gently nudged him and he came around, but the time was just long enough for everyone to realize Charley was staring into space. They all laughed. I will never forget how sad I felt. I wanted to tell them Charley had a seizure, but didn't because revealing his epilepsy to total strangers would have embarrassed him much worse than the laughter. My heavy heart wondered how many times my husband had been humiliated from this type of laughter and not known what he had done. If you see someone staring please do not assume they are an idiot or laugh at them. People who have epilepsy can frequently have staring seizures.

Another type of seizure we endured is called an **atonic seizure** where sudden loss of muscle control causes a person to fall. Charley had these seizures often and usually lost bladder control when they occurred. All of our family and friends, at one time or another, witnessed these seizures. We heard Charley making a noise behind us as he slid down a wall or pushed something over he had tried to steady himself with. After resting for a few minutes he recovered though his speech and balance were always affected and he had a headache. I carried extra clothes for Charley, especially if we were going to be away from home. Stay aware of the sudden fall factor. These seizures are unpredictable but I almost learned how to predict them. I only had to be too far away from Charley to catch him and down he would fall.

Charley's hands and arms were affected by seizures called **myoclonic seizures**, or jerks. These seizures are distinguished by brief, forceful jerks which can affect the whole body or just a part. The jerking can be severe enough to make the person fall but I do not remember Charley ever falling. The seizures are brief but frustrating. Charley was lucid when these seizures occurred and the jerking scared him. He tried to force his body to stop jerking but could not. There is a huge accident factor that accompanies these seizures. Myoclonic seizures occurred when Charley was carrying on normally. One time he was setting glass plates on the table and had a myoclonic seizure. I heard glass banging together and turned to see what he was doing. Plate in each hand, Charley watched his arms jerk and make the plates directly crash into each other. The noise sounded like he was trying to destroy every dish we owned. He saw the effect of the seizures and tried to stop jerking but could not get control. The jerking stopped as quickly as it had started and the plates were spared. I told Charley I could always predict these seizures; he only needed to be carrying an item made of glass in each hand and they would begin.

Some behaviors of **simple partial or complex partial** seizures were slight shaking, tooth grinding, sweating, drooling, lip smacking and picking at clothes or skin. Simple partial seizures are activity that occurs in just part of the brain. The symptoms depend on the area of the brain affected. Medical papers state the person does not know when these seizures occur but that is not always true. There were many times that Charley knew he was having a simple partial seizure and he fought with all the power his brain had to make it stop. Grab a wash cloth and wipe the sweat from the person's face and speak soothing words. Look into their eyes, rub their hands and try to connect with them on an inner level. That person is as much in the room when the seizure occurs as they were two seconds before the seizure began.

Other symptoms of simple partial seizures can be twitching, dizziness, numbness, or nausea. At times Charley's hearing, smell, vision and taste were disturbed or out of balance. He had these symptoms but simple partials affected his speech and coordination most often. He mixed up words, such as calling water glass or cars suckers or ice cream soup. Other types of behaviors can manifest from simple partial seizures, some being headaches and exhaustion. Charley's mind tired and he became frustrated from trying to correct and understand himself. Sometimes we got a lot of amusement and laughter from these seizures forcing new words out of his mouth that we had never heard.

Unless you tune into the person who has epilepsy many simple partial seizure symptoms will not be noticed. If they are displaying constant simple partial symptoms then they are having constant seizures. Study the normal and clue into abnormal to judge the level of seizure control you both are dealing with.

I do not know if distinct seizures correlated with some of Charley's other bodily reactions that the constant misfiring neurons in his brain caused. Sometimes the skin on his face tightened and had a gray hue. Occasionally his left eyelid suddenly drooped much like that of a stroke victim and he instantly had a severe headache. Another extremely miserable change Charley suffered with as he aged was for his body to become horribly cold during tonic-clonic seizure events. He shook with cold even when he was in a warm room and wrapped in blankets.

Each person enduring seizures is an individual and each seizure is as individual as the person. There is not one suggestion concerning seizure care that will encompass every circumstance. When Charley began having seizures neither of us could understand our role in life. We walked many unfamiliar paths as we accepted and coped with his illness. I learned no matter how hard I tried there was no way I was going to do everything right. Charley learned that the things seizures robbed us of were not his fault and the losses we suffered were not because he had done anything wrong.

As you seek knowledge about seizures learn to trust yourself. Put your mistakes behind you. Always look forward and focus on all you are doing right because you have endured and are willing to continually learn. That really is how you live with seizures: endure and learn.

Chapter 2
Adjusting to Epilepsy

O ne of the goals for this book is to help everyone affected by epilepsy to understand how difficult epilepsy is for the person who has seizures. I create scenarios within this chapter that your eyes read but your brain cannot compute. Read the imagined scenarios, become a bit brain scrambled and try to understand living with constantly misfiring neurons as if you were the person who has epilepsy.

What would life be like if we had to train our brains to use our senses differently? For instance if we listened with our noses instead of our ears? Suppose our ears contained the sense of smell and not our nose. Can you imagine asking another person to smell something with their right ear and see if the scent is different than their left ear determined?

Suppose our tongues contained our eyes and we had to open our mouths to see. Then we could tell each other to shut our mouths and quit looking! What if we had to learn to poke food into our eye sockets because that is where our taste buds were? If our bodies were changed instantly, each of these scenarios true, and we were forced to retrain our brains to relay proper signals to each of our senses how would we fare?

Imagine the difficulty in having to change our brain signals and the way our bodies have always functioned in order to survive. How much time would we waste wishing for our old bodies to return because staying with the old is so much easier than adjusting to the new? It takes intense thinking to force the brain to readjust its signals. Correctly directing readjusted signals to each body part and functioning normally would be very challenging.

Everyone knows we are not going to have our senses switched. But, can you state which body part in my made up scenarios switched and had the sense of smell, vision, taste, and hearing without having to go back and look over the former paragraphs? I had to reread as I wrote to keep up with the imaginary sensory switches because my brain would not grasp the thoughts I was trying to force it to process. Our brains know the ears hear, nose smells, eyes see and the tongue tastes. Imaginarily trying to switch our thought patterns concerning our senses scrambles our signals. Tell your brain the ears sense fragrances and the nose hears and your brain will not accept the input or process the thought. Give your brain the signal to tell your nose to stop listening. Instruct your brain to tell your tongue to not look and tell your brain to make your ears sniff. Your brain will not process those thoughts.

Welcome to the world of epilepsy where many misunderstood people live. In this world accurate input to the brain sometimes scrambles and produces inaccurate output often resulting in seizures, scrambled thoughts, misstated words and misunderstood actions. Subtle changes in brain signals can create odd thoughts, actions and behaviors on a daily, hourly, or minute by minute basis. There is no guidance system for comprehending the problems and misunderstanding epilepsy creates.

Adjusting to having epilepsy is not easy. Charley's concentration was consumed with trying to keep his signals straight. A person who has epilepsy learns not to take their thoughts for granted and expect instant cooperation between brain signals and body actions. Though Charley laughed about many of the situations epilepsy created he often fell into the grumbler category as he adjusted to having epilepsy because he hated the damage seizures did and the changes constantly forced upon him. At times he cried and some days was angry beyond any reasoning for all that epilepsy took from him. But he never quit. Charley complained but never let the forced adjustments of epilepsy rob him of his talents or take away his joy of achievement.

If you have epilepsy set goals and be proud of your accomplishments. Dig within yourself, find your survival instincts and use them to flourish. Don't fault yourself for bad days and don't let bad days turn into bad weeks. The more you are thankful for the less you concentrate on the things that epilepsy has unfairly taken away.

Don't quit if you are adjusting to having epilepsy or expect a big change in everyone around you because they cannot completely understand. Those of us who live with someone who has epilepsy can only try to comprehend your trials and tribulations. Everyone's lessons are learned by trial and error.

Epilepsy forces a person to look at the world with new eyes. Do not let epilepsy surround you in darkness and steal your vision. Seek out everything life has to offer and enjoy. It is alright to grumble and cry while adjusting but it is not healthy to hold a grudge against life because of epilepsy. We did not like living with Charley's epilepsy but kept moving forward. Our life was not perfect but we made our sacrifices, adjusted and tried to see life anew every day.

The good news, for anyone who has epilepsy, is you do not have to breath with your ears, hear with your nose, chew with your eyeballs or see with your tongue. But, like Charley, you may have to use one hand to steady the other when you are shaky. Other people might have to drive you places in order to keep the world safe. You may call a car a frizzle-frazzle or a boat a glitch or other things by the wrong name and wonder why everyone else in the room doesn't understand what you are saying. You may start looking for a hammer and come back to your project with a saw and have to ask someone what tool you were needing. You might lose your newspaper when it was just in your hand. You could forget taking a measurement and not realize you had already written it until you are writing it beside the first.

You may change the tire on your boat trailer and forget to tighten the lug nuts and not realize the wheel is loose until it pops off the trailer and runs you a close race down the highway. You might pull your boat trailer up a steep mountain, back into the water, unload the boat, and upon unhooking the trailer realize the ball has no nut on the bottom and the trailer could have easily been next on the "guess what passed me on the highway today" list. You may not be thinking straight and innocently try to burn a small pile of grass without having a water hose handy and burn several acres of your neighbors land before the fire department can respond. You might rebel about not driving and have a seizure while driving and land your car in the top of some pretty tall trees on the side of the road before willingly relinquishing your driver's license. You may take your boat on the lake and forget to put the plug in and be too stubborn to admit the boat is filling with water until the water is splashing up over your feet.

You may unknowingly make inappropriate statements that hurt people you would never hurt intentionally and have to live with the unfair consequences of their not understanding all the negative aspects of your epilepsy. You may find yourself crying for no reason or reprimanded for laughing at situations that are not funny but for some reason your laugher kicked in at the wrong time. You may have to be carried out of many doors you walked into on your own only moments before.

There are many difficult adjustments a person who has epilepsy and their family have to make. Expect disappointments and a great deal of misunderstanding. At times the heartache consumes everyone. A person who has epilepsy is cheated out of much and given very little. The life-long changes epilepsy creates are worth the work it takes to adjust. Charley had severe epilepsy and I know he would say every adjustment was worth the effort. He fulfilled many dreams and accomplished every important goal that he set in life. One of those goals was to stop having seizures. Twenty-four years after setting that goal Charley had his left temporal lobe removed and never had another seizure. Another of those goals was to build our home and he did, settling for no less than the two story house he had dreamed of building and living in since childhood.

If you are adjusting to epilepsy find some grit and work toward accomplishing your dreams. Set goals and meet some every day. Regardless of the losses epilepsy creates the illness cannot take away your pride or determination unless you let it.

Seizures sometimes will steal your body.
Do not ever allow seizures to steal your soul.

Chapter 3
I am a Carpenter

I used to joke with Charley and tell him I was going to make him wear a big padded blow-up suit when I suspected he was going to have seizures. I threatened to roll him around the house and to the car and stuff him in the trunk if we went anywhere. I guarantee if he had worn that suit twenty-three out of twenty-four hours a day the one hour he was unprotected would have been when a seizure occurred. I could usually tell within days of Charley having seizures that he was due an episode but there was no way to know exactly when. Life was so unpredictable.

Initially Charley's seizures scared me and I called for an ambulance every time they occurred. Eventually I stopped panicking and learned how to take care of him and did not call for help unless he had non-stop seizures. If he did not regain enough consciousness to be able to swallow oral medication he had to be given intravenous drugs to get the seizures under control.

I also called for an ambulance when Charley injured himself due to seizures and I could not assess the extent of the injuries. I did not like calling for help in either situation because it placed Charley in the hands of strangers who were professional medical staff but often had never actually witnessed a seizure and did not understand the after-effects.

The ambulance rides and resulting hospital stays introduced Charley to a lot of strangers that asked too many questions as far as he was concerned. He was uncomfortable with the questions because he had no memory of his seizure. One minute he might be in our living room and the next wake up in a hospital emergency room nose to nose with a doctor as he held Charley's eyelid open with one hand and shined a flashlight in his eye with the other.

Charley's seizures originated in his left temporal lobe which also contained his speech center. After a seizure he could not talk until his brain unscrambled but he was always questioned by the medical staff so they could measure how coherent he was. As he regained consciousness he answered most of the questions correctly and satisfied the staff that his mind was sound. Inevitably, someone always asked Charley if he was an epileptic and his firm answer was always, "No, I am a carpenter." Charley was a carpenter who happened to have seizures who absolutely refused to be called an epileptic.

Charley felt being labeled an epileptic created the potential for seizures to take over his identity. He never understood why epilepsy carried a label that implied he is a product of the illness (an epileptic) rather than specifying that he was a person who suffered from what the illness caused (seizures). There are many limits placed upon the life of a person who has seizures. Considering oneself to be a product of their illness is not a limit anyone should ever accept. Charley never gave his identity over to epilepsy. Seizures did not stop him unless they knocked him to the ground, and even then he was quick to get up and start again.

My Charley was a talented carpenter with rough hands, a strong heart and undefeatable determination. If you have epilepsy refuse to be labeled. Be everything you want and do not settle for being an epileptic just because you are a person who happens to have seizures.

Chapter 4

We Never Have Tomorrow

I read a letter to Dear Abby from a woman that was in love with a man who had epilepsy whose family did not want her to marry him because of his illness. The woman asked Abby for an opinion and she replied that many people with epilepsy live a normal life and the epilepsy should not be the deciding factor of whether a person will make a good marriage partner. I agree with Abby.

When I initially read the letter my thought was that someone needs to tell that lady if she marries a person who has epilepsy she will not be able to count on having tomorrow. I was surprised that idea immediately came to mind. I never before had contemplated our tomorrows being stolen by seizures.

Throughout years of living with epilepsy Charley's illness worsened and abilities became limited. We slowly, unknowingly conditioned ourselves to not count on tomorrow because today's were cancelled by seizures so we learned to take advantage of every minute of every today. When Charley was not having seizures we worked together on projects and maintenance when his thoughts were processing normally. As time progressed he could not take of care anything without my help. The more his brain tormented him the weaker his body became (don't take this sentence lightly. A brain exhausted by seizures will eventually cause a body to be weak).

At the end of a day of routine maintenance most people can stop and plan on working the next day. We stopped working on our projects but could not plan on the next day. Charley often had seizures before our projects were finished which cost us tomorrow and the ability to complete tasks together. The burden fell upon me to complete work alone.

If you can count on tomorrow you are very lucky. Without tomorrow days can become long. If you are planning to be the companion of a person who might not have tomorrow be willing to learn to complete tasks alone so if seizures do steal today you are prepared.

One time Charley and I began replacing a water line to our house and he had a seizure which marked the end of his day. The water was turned off, pipe cut in half, and my husband lying on top of our tools snoring as he slept off the seizure. These occasions frustrated me tremendously but I had no choice but to roll Charley off the tools and finish. People who have epilepsy walk a very fine line. Jobs must be completed and tasks accomplished but exhaustion can cause seizures. You won't find an easy answer to making sense of life with epilepsy.

Our experiences taught us by trial and error. If the person who has epilepsy feels on the edge of seizures do not begin a crucial project. Stay busy with a project or hobby that can be completed in spurts. Begin time-consuming projects only on good days. We kept a maintenance list that we checked and then decided what to tackle depending on how Charley felt. Plans backfired and seizures stole our days but I managed. Call friends or family for backup before you begin projects and make sure they can help you finish projects if seizures occur.

You will find planning around potential seizures frustrating but do not push the person who has epilepsy into working when your instincts tell you they don't feel well. They are constantly fighting a battle to keep their brain waves straight which creates a need for more time to successfully complete tasks. Though Charley needed extra time, after mentally planning a job he finished projects if seizures did not knock him down.

If you are the companion of someone who has epilepsy learn how to do alone what you expect to do together. I do not know how many occasions, sometimes laughing and others crying, that I rolled a snoozing Charley off of our tools after he had an unexpected seizure.

Acknowledge the potential loss of tomorrow as a cold hard fact of epilepsy. Facts eliminate fear. If you are afraid of everything that seizures may cause then epilepsy has you instead of you having epilepsy. Never let epilepsy have you!

Helping someone you love with every aspect of their illness makes your heart feel very full. Sitting alone wishing your companion was awake instead of sleeping off seizures makes your heart feel very empty. Enjoy life when you have today and find contentment when seizures steal your tomorrows.

Chapter 5
Within the Public Realm

Consideration for people who have seizures has not improved much since we began living with epilepsy in 1980. There are many stumbling blocks for people with epilepsy when they venture out in public. Laws regarding accommodating individuals with disabilities should also encompass assistance and understanding for people who have seizures.

For instance, warning signs in loud and suddenly flashy establishments would be helpful. Charley and I tried to avoid those places because that environment caused seizures. We could not attend carnivals because of the blinking lights and noisy crowds but we knew that. Learn what atmospheres might cause seizures and avoid them if possible.

The public has a need for artificial stimulation which people with epilepsy do not need. Seizures cause millions of brain neurons to backfire randomly and that provides plenty of stimulation. I never intentionally took Charley to an atmosphere that was bursting with artificial stimulation, but due to a lack of warning signs we found it impossible to completely avoid them.

A friend of ours (not a very bright friend, they knew Charley had seizures) recommended a restaurant on our twentieth wedding anniversary. We went to the restaurant and upon entering saw no warning signs or reasons to be alarmed about the atmosphere. We were seated at a table in the middle of the restaurant enjoying our conversation and the lights were suddenly turned off and dozens of different colors of bright flashing lights that were placed on the ceiling started randomly blinking.

Charley's brain was overworking as he adjusted to the public atmosphere. The flashing lights overloaded him and created instant misery. He covered his eyes and screamed like he was being murdered. I ran to a restaurant employee and asked him to please turn off the flashing lights explaining that my husband had epilepsy. The employee grudgingly complied, but turning off the lights left us in a restaurant full of unhappy non-artificially stimulated people who had expected to see a table dance (we later found out). We were the only people who had a problem with the flashing lights.

The other people were eating at that restaurant because they enjoyed the flashing lights and loud atmosphere. We had no idea that environment existed. Our food was ordered and we chose to stay but the rest of the evening was awkward. I probably should of called the restaurant and inquired about the atmosphere prior to eating there but really, no one should have to go to that extreme in order to interact with the public.

A warning sign such as "Please inform an employee if you have epilepsy and we will not turn on the flashing lights" placed at the entrance to the restaurant would have given us a fair chance. People who suffer from seizures might be happy with "go away if you have epilepsy" at this point. I would have found another restaurant rather than have Charley tormented had I been given an option. I hope in the future public awareness of many aspects of epilepsy skyrockets. Signs that offer help to seizure patients or warning of randomly flashing lights and sudden extreme noise levels would be excellent.

Another aspect of dealing with the public realm was seizures happening in unpredictable places and strangers panicking. When we were grocery shopping and the cart began to unexpectedly roll behind me I knew Charley was pushing the cart forward or sideways as he fell. When we were at the checkout lane of a store and Charley was in front of me and I saw the cashier's eyes grow gigantic as they looked at him, I knew he was beginning to have a seizure. When Charley went into an establishment and he took a while and I heard sirens in the distance, I knew he was having a seizure. When he left home with friends and I answered the phone and heard a hysterical person, I knew Charley was having a seizure. When he was working outside and later came in the house and I noticed dirt all over his clothes and grass stuck in his hair, I knew Charley had a seizure. When I sent him with various items to put away in the garage and later saw the items lying scattered in the yard and no Charley to be found, I knew he was wondering around after having had a seizure. When I came downstairs in the mornings and discovered myself surrounded by broken glass in the kitchen floor, I knew a seizure had occurred sometime during the night.

When Charley was not with me I could tell when he had a seizure so I certainly knew he had a seizure when we were together in public. Nice people usually braved the unknown and offered to help when Charley had fallen. Total strangers supported one side of him and I held on to the other as we walked him to our vehicle. Most people are nice and they mean well, but even nice people in the public realm tend to panic and make unnecessary mistakes when seizures occur. These mistakes often cause the seizure patient and their caretakers more problems than having a seizure does.

Charley helped my brother David, who owns a restaurant, deliver caterings. That was a great way for Charley to work without having to drive. He enjoyed being around people and got out of the house. Charley used to shake his head and say he never imagined having to trade his hammer for a cook pot. He never expected life would force him to change from being a full-time carpenter to a part-time caterer. Charley was quite famous around our small town. For years people had known him as David's hardworking brother-in-law but did not know he had epilepsy. They were shocked to unexpectedly witness Charley's seizures but formed a great respect and admiration for him because he refused to let those seizures stop his life.

One Thanksgiving Charley and I were helping David deliver a catering to the third floor of a bank. I was exiting the foyer after hauling the first load of food. David was outside the bank with Charley walking behind him carrying a tray that held six pumpkin pies. David was rolling a cart that had an insulated bag full of food and a five gallon bucket of tea on it. As I began to exit the foyer doors I looked at Charley and immediately knew he was beginning to have a seizure and was slowly falling down face first. The tray of pumpkin pies he was carrying began to precariously tumble forward and pass David in the air as Charley lost his balance. The pies flew past David who then realized Charley was having a seizure. David clumsily grabbed at Charley as he fell forward in an attempt to help with his landing. The bucket of tea was shoved off the cart by the two of them and poured down the sidewalk.

There David and I stood with Charley lying on the ground having a mild seizure. David gathered the scattered pumpkin pies while I took care of Charley. Though the pies were scrambled they landed in the pans and were ugly, but edible. The lid to the bucket of tea had been knocked several feet away and the tea was slowly streaming down the sidewalk.

People checked on us but no one seemed panicked. David went upstairs while I got my Charley back on his feet and took him to the company van and sat him in the passenger seat. He could not talk but did comprehend what I was saying. I told him, "I am going to help David set the catering and then we will go make more tea." Charley nodded so I knew he understood. I then said, "You sit your ass in this van and do not get out or open the door for any reason." Charley nodded. He lost bladder control when the seizure occurred but was not lucid enough to realize his pants were wet. I was afraid he might come stumbling upstairs and try to help us with the catering when he regained any ability to walk. I was very firm and said again, "You keep your ass in this van." Charley nodded. I quickly kissed him and went into the bank to help David set the catering.

Some of the people at the catering had experienced Charley's seizures previously so they understood the situation and told us not to worry about how the pie looked. As David was setting the catering he walked past the window and looked out and craned his neck as he tried to process what he was seeing. Then he said, "Good Lord, Lola, you had better get down there quick."

I ran over and peered down on the parking lot and nearly fell over. Two fire trucks and an ambulance were parked next to the van. Emergency lights were flashing lighting up the entire parking lot. A fireman was at the driver's side of the van and an ambulance attendant the other, both loudly knocking on the windows trying to get Charley to open the door. He was not able to talk but he knew I told him to keep his ass in the van and not open the door for any reason. Charley sure kept his ass in the van and that door was not coming open until I returned. I quickly made my way to the parking lot and explained to the emergency workers that Charley would be fine.

"Who called an ambulance?" I asked the paramedic.

"A bystander." the paramedic answered. A good-hearted person who saw our catastrophe and thought we needed help. When Charley was lying on the ground I told the people who inquired about him that we did not need an ambulance. Apparently someone thought differently.

If you are a bystander witnessing a person have a seizure please do not immediately call an ambulance. Go to the caretaker, if the person having the seizure is not alone, and ask if an ambulance is needed. Only if they request an ambulance should one be called. A huge problem created by having seizures in public is caused by good intentioned people who do not know what is happening calling an ambulance.

If you choose to help a person who has had a seizure please remember you are a total stranger and their brain is in a disoriented crisis situation. Charley grabbed more than one terrified stranger by the shirt and trapped them against his chest because he was confused. Be prepared to quickly get out of the reach of a person who has just had a seizure. Stay calm and do not shout, repeatedly ask their name or question them. Be comforting, kind and calmly reassuring. Give their brain time to recover (at least fifteen to twenty minutes minimum) and allow conversation to flow at their pace.

Everyone dealing with epilepsy wishes for greater education and public awareness regarding seizures. The unjust fear factor hanging over seizures, and the people who have them, needs to be eliminated. The situation will not improve until society is ready to open their minds and examine the inner aspects of living with epilepsy. Lack of knowledge concerning seizures is what has created the fear of epilepsy society holds on to so adeptly. This fear is cast onto the people who suffer from seizures creating the reverse of what society should provide in order to adequately meet the seizure patient's needs.

If you are a person who has seizures or their caretaker get out into the world. Don't be ashamed of seizures. How are people who are unfamiliar with epilepsy supposed to understand when seizures are hidden behind closed doors? Hundreds of people saw Charley have a seizure at one time or another because we did not hide them. His psychotic behavior did thrust us behind closed doors but that is a different chapter.

If you were afraid of people who have seizures and had no

knowledge about epilepsy before, I hope you now know if you see someone having a seizure . . . run toward them . . . and not away.

Chapter 6

The Medical Community

Protecting a person who has seizures creates an inner radar system within their caretaker. I was always on the lookout for hazards. One place Charley received medical care was at the Veteran's Hospital. A few years ago the front of the hospital was remodeled and a huge revolving door installed. The door slowly turns in a circle as visitors step into a large slot between glass panels to enter the hospital. I hated that door and am astounded that someone actually designed and others agreed to install such a door as a hospital entrance. On each side of the revolving door are two hinged glass doors that remain locked. Every time we stepped into our revolving door slot I was afraid that Charley would have a seizure and the door would hurt him. I wondered if the door's gears might start smoking and a motor melt if his body kept it from revolving. I was not strong enough to drag him out if he became trapped within the glass walls. I worried if he had a seizure other people might be trapped in their revolving door slots.

A revolving door with no other options for the main entrance of a hospital was the type of obstacle my radar always honed in on. That door was a danger and one of many we faced daily. The perfect example of a potential hazard created by a lack of knowledge regarding seizure patient's needs is the staff of a medical facility not realizing someone might have a seizure and instantly fall while inside one of those door slots. Keep the side doors unlocked please!

We encountered various obstacles within the medical community while dealing with seizures. I am sure many "seizure people" can name at least one hospital rule that could not be broken prior to a seizure occurring. When Charley had a seizure the unbreakable rules quickly flew out the window in order to reunite us.

On several occasions Charley had to have routine medical tests and it was never in his best interest to be alone during these tests because he became very emotional. I am sure some people who have epilepsy probably can undergo routine tests while alone but Charley needed me. If I was with him we usually prevented a seizure. I explained to medical technicians that being alone while undergoing tests scrambled Charley. My requests to accompany him almost always fell upon deaf ears. Usually the technician stood solidly in front of me, arms crossed, and positively forbid me to enter the forbidden area. Before letting Charley leave I always asked who would take care of him if he had a seizure.

"I will." every technician stated, and off they went. When Charley's emotions were on overload I could almost count to the second the time it would take before he began to have a seizure.

On numerous occasions as I sat in the waiting room, the same technician who had promised to take care of my husband ran past me while frantically scanning the room trying to locate me because Charley had a seizure. Eventually the technician saw me quietly staring at them and told me I was needed in the forbidden area. I am puzzled with regulations that ignore the emotional aspects of epilepsy. I could not guarantee the absence of a seizure if I was with Charley but I provided a sense of security that helped him withstand situations without unnecessarily stirring up his emotions.

When Charley had seizures he was confused and lost while recovering but stayed calm if I was nearby. If I was not present he scared medical personnel half to death by grabbing them and pulling them down on top of his chest and not letting go. That was simply Charley's way of saying, "go get my wife." Believe me, his method worked every time. When I was allowed in the forbidden areas of the hospital Charley sensed my presence and released the terrified technician. The captured person and I eventually laughed together about the incident. I was sorry they were scared silly but they could not deny the warning I had given them. Charley never would have grabbed them if I had been in the room. I did not understand putting the seizure patient or medical staff through such trauma. If you are the caregiver of a person who has seizures and you know they need you present more than the medical facility needs to follow petty rules attempt to get them to make an exception. If enough people who deal with seizures prove their case perhaps some unnecessary rules can be changed. It is time to respect the emotional needs of seizure patients and allow their companions to accompany them during routine medical tests when possible.

I have been scoffed at while trying to protect Charley and advise medical staff of the severity and spontaneity of his seizures, but usually only once. I was on a first name basis with many nurses and technicians and never became angry when not allowed to accompany my husband. I always hoped the raw fear Charley caused by grabbing and trapping them had taught a lesson of respect for future seizure patients' needs. It was sad that it took Charley suffering a seizure before the staff allowed me into the forbidden areas.

The medical community needs to trust the caregiver or partner of the person with epilepsy and ask what is best for the patient. In dealing with seizures we need to stop relying on what can only be seen through the eyes of medical equipment. That equipment does not show a tenth of the complexities within a misfiring brain. Regard each patient as an individual with separate needs and see if the world falls apart if a few rules are broken.

As the years rolled on Charley's seizures and hospital visits became more frequent. I had to set limits with the medical community in order to protect him. The following paragraphs talk about several common mistakes I have seen.

Some of Charley's nurses were my friends so I know this was not intentional but I have seen him treated as if having a seizure creates instant deafness. Do not yell at a person recuperating from a seizure. The first question most medical personnel ask someone after a seizure is "what is your name?" Loudly speaking "what is your name" to the person who has had a seizure is not going to make them speak their name sooner. Charley's lack of an answer was because his seizure activity was located in the speech area of his brain. The lack of a sensible answer does not mean the person who just had a seizure cannot hear.

I hope this is an outdated concept but just in case: If I am wrong shoot me, but I have taken care of Charley during hundreds of seizures and have never once seen him swallow his tongue. I did not allow anyone to stick an instrument into his mouth because it always did more harm than good. Many years ago I was instructed by doctors to hold Charley's tongue down when he had a seizure and given a soft plastic curved instrument for the purpose. The only time something can be poked in the mouth of a person having a seizure is at the initial onset of the seizure. If you manage to get an instrument poked into the mouth it is nearly impossible to keep the seizure patient's lips off of the instrument before the teeth clamp shut. The person with the instrument is trying to hold down the tongue and not paying attention to the lips of the patient (believe me, I know this from experience with many seizures). When an instrument is slid into the patient's mouth the bottom lip is dry and tends to stick to the instrument. Then the lip rolls over the bottom teeth and is wedged between the instrument and the teeth. The mouth clamps shut and the lip is chewed to pieces during the seizure, which is unnecessary and extremely painful. Do not poke anything into the mouth of a person who is having a seizure.

Another thing I observed with the obsession to keep the seizure patient from swallowing their tongue is the person attempting to wedge the instrument between the teeth by force. Even when having a seizure Charley's brain registered enough to know someone was pushing against him trying to force something into his mouth and he became very combative. My main concerns were to keep him safe and make sure he recovered from the seizure with dignity. I always grabbed a urinal first to contain the loss of bladder control. It is difficult to roll a person who is having a seizure on their side and catch their urine while someone else is trying to force an instrument into their mouth.

I learned (not as soon as I should have) to forbid anyone from poking any instrument (including a tongue depressor) in Charley's mouth when he began to have a seizure. When told Charley might die from swallowing his tongue my answer was, "Let him." I preferred that more than him waking up with a bloody, swollen, chewed-to-pieces lip and having to answer to why I allowed someone to cause him unnecessary pain. I sincerely hope the idea of a person swallowing their tongue while having a seizure is over forever.

Epilepsy is an individual illness with a personality of its own that fits no mold. If you are the caretaker or companion of someone with epilepsy protect them and demand the respect you both deserve. Never assume medical staff know a fraction of what you do about seizures or the person you love.

Of the hundreds of medical personnel that Charley and I knew not one of them would tell you I was ever rude. I respected the medical staff for their vast knowledge in areas I knew nothing about. I constantly tried to increase my knowledge about seizures and never felt I could learn if I made enemies of the teachers. I learned a lot about epilepsy from medical personnel throughout the years. I think they learned a lot about epilepsy from Charley and I.

Chapter 7

The Strength of the Mind

Physical seizures are not the only battle a person with epilepsy has. Epilepsy would be simple if it only consisted of having seizures and sleeping until their effects pass. Charley fought a battle in his mind that was invisible to everyone. I doubt we are the only people who have lived with the unseen battles the strong mind of a person who has epilepsy fights.

People from all walks in life can relate to common struggles. The understanding Charley received from others was grounded in a comprehension of the mutual problems of society. Having epilepsy made his life something others could not comprehend. Anyone suffering with seizures needs more understanding because of the strength their minds are forced to use to survive.

There was something in Charley's brain, I wish I could explain it (misfiring neurons?) that was constantly pulling him. As this something was pulling he was pushing back in order to keep his thoughts and actions on an even keel. Most people have no clue this battle exists. I tuned in to Charley to help him maintain equalization between the mind battles that tortured him and his outer character that had no chance of appearing normal. His words were often spoken harshly because he could not push away something that was pulling within his brain and constantly maintain normal mannerisms.

Before I understood Charley's brain battles we sometimes argued because of the tone of his statements. He claimed I misinterpreted his words and I unknowingly had. I eventually realized he expressed emotions the best he could for someone who had thousands of neurons misfiring in his brain's speech center. I did not see those neurons misfiring through a visible seizure and I had unfair expectations of him. The gradual increase in intensity of this mental war in combination with hundreds of seizures wore Charley's mind down. I wish I had recognized the struggle within his brain sooner and left him alone when he needed space. One day when Charley was frustrated because I had misunderstood the meaning of his words he wrote, "The personality of one is not the personality of what one sees from the inside." I did my best to understand Charley and tried to be patient and loving. He accomplished so much in spite of epilepsy. I resented unfair circumstances epilepsy caused but I did not begrudge Charley his illness. He fought with all the strength his mind had to accomplish simple tasks most people could do with no mental exertion. Epilepsy extremes are not because of a weak mind. They are the result of a strong mind fighting a battle that no one can explain. Electrical impulses misfiring sounds simple but you will learn there is nothing simple about epilepsy.

The worse days of Charley's brain battles were evident by signs of extreme agitation with no visible seizures. I learned to leave him alone and not try to talk about the problem. When these battles were raging I could not improve the situation. I was frustrated but understood that Charley was unable to fix these struggles. Intervening when someone is pushing against their brain that is pulling away is like trying to break up a dog fight. Step in the middle of two dogs fighting and you are going to get bit.

When Charley was fighting his mental battles I visualized him and his brain struggling about ten feet away from the edge of a cliff. Charley pushed and his brain pulled and then Charley pulled and his brain pushed. Day by day, hour by hour, or minute by minute they slowly inched closer and closer to the edge of the cliff. During those times Charley was using the strength of his mind for all it was worth as he mentally pushed seizures away; fighting the battle but never winning the war. Eventually seizures resulted and Charley and his brain both fell over the cliff. In spite of seizures I am convinced that people who have epilepsy are mentally some of the strongest people in the world.

When we care for someone and know them as individuals we discover and accept their disabilities. Accepting the inabilities of others helps us know ourselves as individuals, thus determining our strength of character and the true depth of our abilities. If someone you love has seizures take the time to observe and know them. Recognize and build who you are by learning and accepting who they are not.

Chapter 8

Sheltering Charley

You will find trying to maintain another person's individuality and keeping their dignity intact is one of the greatest obstacles that epilepsy creates for a caretaker. In any relationship each person's dignity is preserved by their ability to maintain a separate individuality. Sustaining the status of individuals when one person is caretaker and the other dependant upon that caretaker is very difficult. In our seizure relationship I was the protector and Charley the protected.

Charley was a very proud man who accomplished something every day unless he was sick. I tried to maintain his individuality but sometimes do not feel I did the job correctly. I babied Charley and did not allow anyone who did not understand epilepsy to see him on bad days. I was extremely unfriendly to people who visited our home without having made sure we were prepared for company. When unexpected company arrived at our house if Charley was not having seizures he was very welcoming. I was asking them to pick up the telephone and call before arriving at our home while Charley was telling them to stop by any time.

I now realize how funny it was that at the same time Charley could not hide his pleasure in visiting with unexpected company I could not hide my annoyance at their arrival. I tried to be friendly, but my fear of anyone becoming comfortable unexpectedly dropping into our home overrode any ability I had to be nice. Charley did not understand his illness enough to realize I had his best interests at heart. I could not explain my motives because he was not able to see our life from my perspective.

If you know someone who has seizures call them before visiting. Make sure they are not having seizures and unable to visit. My stress level would have been greatly reduced if others had extended this common courtesy. Caretakers of someone who has seizures – firmly establish the boundary with others of picking up the telephone and calling or emailing before visiting to make sure your day is fit for company.

Unexpected company arriving at our home when Charley was having seizures created problems. People who have never dealt with epilepsy have no clue the watch a caretaker must maintain. When Charley had a seizure and others were present I was observed running to get a urinal, unzipping his pants and aiming his penis to catch the urine. I never needed an audience for those duties and neither do you. Many times when seizures occurred Charley lost bladder control. All I could do was undress him and cover his naked body with a blanket. When he recovered his last thought was whether or not he was wearing clothes. Anyone at our house at that time sure got to see a naked Charley.

The person you love will never hand you any aspect of their personality and say, "Here, this is no longer mine." On some occasions you will unknowingly try to take over their individuality. On those occasions listen to their protests and respect the fact that they have the right to be an individual. Charley fought me tooth and nail when I overstepped his individuality boundaries. My heart hurt terribly when I accidentally bruised his dignity in the process of trying to protect him. I strove to balance my duties and slowly learned a person's dignity cannot be preserved by disallowing them to be an individual.

As I tried to protect Charley's dignity I sacrificed my identity because I became the bad guy. I stopped him from helping others with carpentry projects when I knew they could not take care of him during seizures. Sometimes he loaned tools to friends and forgot. I had to call everyone we knew to find our missing tools. I made Charley quit loaning tools because he worked his mind to a frazzle thinking someone had stolen what actually was borrowed. He did not have the heart to say no to anyone and felt guilty when he did. I told him to tell those who asked to borrow our tools, "Lola will not allow loaning, and you don't have to live with Lola." I became the bad guy to protect Charley from emotional frustration. I don't regret having been the bad guy to protect my husband, but I hated being misunderstood. In the process of trying to overcome different obstacles that epilepsy creates you will stumble and have to deal with actions of your own that even you don't understand. That is a part of learning the life of epilepsy so don't be too hard on yourself.

Another major stumbling block we encountered with Charley's individuality issues was being forced to surrender his drivers license to the State of Texas after a seizure occurred while he was driving (he had a wreck that should have been on Nascar). We could not deny he was a danger. Charley knew the time had come to stop driving but losing his independence was heart breaking. I didn't have to worry that he might have a seizure while driving, but I was not glad he had to surrender his license.

A person's dignity is very fragile. Charley's loss of driving privileges and relying on others for transportation was a huge affront on his dignity that placed a heavy burden on me. We dealt with this the best we could, along with all the other unexpected obstacles epilepsy threw in front of us. Charley did not like depending on me to supply his every need. We live ten miles from the nearest hardware store, which left him in limbo as he worked on projects because he could not obtain needed items. He grudgingly waited for me to get supplies but his memory was terrible. Often we returned home from the hardware store after buying materials and he had forgotten the first thing needed in order to begin a project. We had many "how on earth could you forget that?" occasions. Grumbling to myself, I returned and bought the forgotten items. These situations reminded Charley that I carried more than my fair share because of his epilepsy and that bothered him immensely. If you are having to carry a heavy load because someone you love has seizures try to gain a fair perspective on whose burdens weigh more. You can drive, they cannot. You can work, often they cannot. You can walk without the constant fear of falling, they cannot. The list is endless. Use that list frequently in order to be thankful and not bitter.

If your dignity is wounded and life seems unfair because you cannot drive due to seizures **<u>DO NOT</u>** give up hope. We never dreamed Charley would drive again, but he did. After brain surgery eliminated seizures, he reapplied for a driver's license. After taking the written test a gazillion times before he remembered the correct answers and passed he was mobile and independent. There is no easy answer as to how to be depended on by a person you love and encourage them to be independent. It is very difficult to be a caregiver for someone and not get into the habit of thinking the choices you make for them must be better than their own.

The most outstanding aspect of Charley's individuality was his talent as a carpenter. He loved improving our home. My favorite method of encouragement was keeping him supplied with projects. We drew plans and enjoyed contemplating preferred designs. After estimating needed materials we went to the hardware store to purchase supplies. We bought extra materials so he did not have to deal with the frustration of not being able to drive. Upon completion of a project Charley's individuality was at the top of its game, pride shining, and dignity always fully intact.

If you have seizures and feel you are losing your individuality find something you like to do and learn to be good at it. Root out your talents and enjoy them. If you feel untalented force yourself to take an interest in something and pursue lessons. Look forward to the finished product. Search until you find a niche that you are happy in. Never quit. Set goals and always strive to finish what you start. Seizures cannot take away your pride or sense of accomplishment unless you let them. If you love or are the caretaker of someone who has seizures work on finding a comfortable way to balance protecting them with promoting their individuality. Helping Charley maintain his individuality as he fought the daily losses seizures created was the right thing to do. I have been told you can love someone too much and if that is true then I am guilty of the charge. In spite of my efforts I never really felt confident that I found the perfect balance to preserving Charley's dignity.

But Charley did,
and he tolerated my mistakes.
For that I loved him dearly.

Clusters of Seizures
and
Postictal Psychosis

The Darker Side
of our Story

As I Emerge

As we go through life some traumatic situations weaken us and others make us stronger, thus forcing us to create different personalities within ourselves. Within us exists one weak and one strong character. When life takes away choices our characters have to learn to live in harmony even though each one is not allowed to interact. If we are consistently strong our weak character is pushed aside and eventually smothered by feelings of strength and determination. The ability to think correctly is lost because our strength takes action before our thoughts allow weakness to emerge. Our strong character dominates while our weak character, though abandoned, is not idle. The weak character observes and waits for a voice. Through the voice of weakness I reveal my strengths.

I loved Charley and was married to him for twenty-six years and had to be strong. I never tried to justify my reasoning for staying married to a person with so many problems. I cursed and prayed and was forced to put away any weak characteristics for the sake of taking care of my husband.

When I began writing this book I did not realize a total stranger lived within me. My weak character has turned out to be the main author of this book. As I tried to recall events my strong character could not remember or explain how I coped. I did not have a clue of my strength until my weak character began to speak within these chapters and reveal how difficult it had been to live within me and not be allowed to exist. I now know what I sacrificed for the sake of another. I have had to find my weak character and bring her back to life in order to remember, write, and cry myself through the memories and trauma of all that Charley and I endured. I have found my tears again.

When I am finished with each chapter I sit and read it out loud. Usually I cry and cry as I read the words that an observant stranger who lived within me has written. Never would the strong me, the great protector of Charley, share such intimate and crushing details of our life. It is the weak character I pushed away for so many years who recalls and writes these words that all of me hopes will find a way to help others.

You would think I could not write until I remember but the opposite is true. I cannot remember until I write. I do not experience the feelings associated with memories until I read each chapter out loud. This book is my way of healing and becoming one person again, someone who is allowed to be both strong and weak. Twenty-six years of knowledge, endurance and strength are represented on these pages. I hope this book helps you as much as it has helped me.

Chapter 9

Clusters of Seizures
and
Postictal Psychosis

The next few chapters are about psychotic behaviors I witnessed that were beyond Charley's control and caused by his epilepsy. They portray a very dark side of our life. Most people who have seizures and those taking care of them will never have to endure these psychotic behaviors. However, recent medical information that is based on ongoing research states that of the 2.5 million Americans who now have epilepsy six to ten percent of them have some degree of psychosis. At least 150,000 to 250,000 people in the United States are battling an invisible illness that has the potential to overcome them if they cannot find any direction or answers to their questions.

I began my journey with Charley's epilepsy and my quest for information in February of 1980. In February of 2011 as I researched medical papers I learned that a metal taste Charley suffered with off and on for more than twenty years was a hallucination. We consulted doctors specifically because this taste was making Charley miserable and no one had an answer. I was astounded while reading about hallucinations to find the answer to Charley's misery thirty-one years after our search began. It is now February of 2012 and recently I found research that says twenty-five to fifty percent of people who have seizures for ten to fifteen years will develop psychosis. There is not enough room in this book to write all the information I have found as I research psychosis and epilepsy.

My website is www.epilepsyunveiled.com. This website will have updates on what information I find about epilepsy, clusters of seizures and psychosis. For those living with psychotic behaviors I write these next chapters because I want you to better understand what you are living with and realize that new information regarding epilepsy and psychosis becomes available every day. Do not give up on your search for information and do not give in to psychosis.

I found three terms relating to psychosis during my research about epilepsy and psychotic behaviors. They are postictal, interictal, and periictal. In Latin the prefix "post" means after or subsequent to. "Ictal" is a word near the Latin word "ictus" which means to strike so "ictal" means seizure or stroke. Postictal (before a strike) Psychosis is commonly believed to happen after seizures (usually tonic-clonic or a series of seizures). The prefix "inter" is a Latin preposition that means between or among. Interictal psychosis occurs between seizures. The term "peri" is a Greek prefix meaning around, about or near-by. Psychosis that develops gradually in parallel with increased seizure frequency is referred to as peri-ictal. Some information I found in medical studies states this psychosis is directly related to epilepsy and irregular discharges in the brain and other research states the opposite (that there is no medical proof that seizures cause this psychosis). These terms are defined to simplify the search for others who are looking for answers in medical research papers.

Charley suffered with psychosis between, before and during seizure episodes. He was medically diagnosed with postictal psychosis and that is the term I use to describe his psychotic behaviors in this book. I have no doubt that every term used to describe psychosis and epilepsy fit Charley at one time or another during his lifetime. At times he was psychotic between rounds of seizures and others before seizures and sometimes after seizures. Other times he had seizures and no signs of psychotic behaviors.

Life is very difficult when you live with a person who has clusters of seizures but do not know what those seizures are, or their potential to create psychosis in an individual. Describing Charley's seizure clusters and psychotic behaviors will help with recognition of this medical phenomenon. If anyone better comprehends their life with seizures after reading about our experiences then I will have met one goal of this book; helping psychotic people and their families understand their illness so they no longer feel lost and alone. The only experience I have with a person who had epilepsy is the twenty-six years Charley and I were together. I am not a doctor or expert in any medical area concerning seizures, psychosis or epilepsy. I write honestly of our life, my observations and information I have found through research.

When you live with a person who is psychotic their bizarre behaviors are evident but it is impossible to grasp their meaning. You can constantly read medical terminology and still not understand enough about the condition to accurately tie the psychotic behaviors you are witnessing to a person's seizures. We are not born with the ability to observe another person's behavior and immediately conclude they are psychotic. The focus of Charley's medical staff was seizures. No doctor ever asked me if Charley was hallucinating or having bizarre thoughts and even if they had I could not have answered correctly. Now I know he was psychotic and had hallucinations. I knew he could not remember anything that had occurred when seizures caused him to be psychotic but who would believe that?

We survived, but lived a hard life. If you are living with this type of epilepsy you need to exist beyond mere survival. I explain Charley's behaviors to help make sense of your situation and give you the confidence to seek help. If you or someone you love has epilepsy and clusters of seizures and psychotic behavior are not a part of your life perhaps our story can be an inspiration. Life can always be worse, even if you do have seizures. If you or someone you love has epilepsy and clusters of seizures are causing psychotic behaviors perhaps our story will be informative and helpful. Life can always be better, even if you do have seizures.

I have read that treatment with the proper antipsychotic medications can avert the psychotic behavior. No treatment is forthcoming if physicians are not informed about the psychotic behavior because the people living with epilepsy do not know what clusters of seizures are, or how to recognize the behaviors they produce. Charley certainly was not capable of telling anyone he was psychotic. I did not know how to describe the behavior but did wonder if psychosis was the culprit wreaking havoc in our life. I hid his behavior thinking no one would believe me if I told them that seizures, on occasion, made my husband irrational, intimidating, and sometimes violent.

There is no question in the medical world that a person who suffers from clusters of seizures can also experience psychosis specifically because of those seizures. Chronic psychosis may develop from recurrent episodes or even a single episode of postictal psychosis. The following are excerpts from a few articles I found:

Epilepsy.com:

"Postictal psychosis has been estimated to affect between 6% and 10% of people with epilepsy. It involves psychiatric symptoms that occur within 7 days (usually within 1 to 3 days) after a seizure or seizure cluster in a person who does not have these symptoms at other times (or at least has them in a much milder form). These symptoms may include delusions, depressive or manic psychosis, or bizarre thoughts and behavior. They generally disappear promptly when treated with low doses of medication."

The Annals of General Psychiatry

"Postictal psychosis (PIP) is characterized by an episode of psychosis occurring within one week after a cluster of seizures. PIP is common. In a study of inpatient video-electroencephalographic monitoring, the annual incidence of postictal psychotic events was estimated to be 6.4% . . . While PIP is usually short-lived, with remission after several days to weeks, chronic psychoses may develop from recurrent episodes or even a single episode . . . psychotic symptoms may include hallucinations, including auditory or visual. Abnormalities of content of thought, such as ideas of reference or delusions (including paranoid, grandiose, somatic, religious, or others) are often present, as may be abnormalities of form of thought."

Epilepsy Currents: Postictal Psychosis: Common, Dangerous, and Treatable written by Orrin Devinsky, M.D.

"Occasionally, after a fit, or, more frequently, after a series of fits, an attack of mental disturbance may come on which lasts for several days. It may be simply a demented state, or there may be hallucinations, with irritability and even violence. Postictal psychosis often complicates chronic epilepsy, especially in patients with seizure clusters that include tonic-clonic seizures, bilateral cerebral dysfunction . . . and a family history of psychiatric illness. Psychosis includes delusions, auditory and visual hallucinations, mood changes, and aggressive behavior. It typically emerges after a lucid interval of hours or days after the last seizure. This treatable disorder is associated with serious morbidity (illness) and mortality (death). Dr. Devinsky has written several medical papers concerning psychosis that can be found on the internet.

After finding information that confirmed my beliefs about Charley's psychosis my next goal was to prove he suffered with clusters of seizures that caused his postictal psychosis. In 2002 Charley was arrested because of a violent episode of psychosis that is explained later in the book. Dr. Diaz-Arrastia (Charley's neurologist) wrote a letter to our district attorney that stated, "Charley had clusters of seizures that caused him to become confused, combative and impulsive with difficulty controlling his emotions and anger outbursts. It is my experience that patients with severe epilepsy frequently experience such severe postictal psychotic behavior problems after clusters of seizures and while they are not usually a danger to anybody but themselves the abnormal behavior frequently brings them to trouble with the law." I had completely forgotten about this letter until I began researching information for this book. Understanding clusters of seizures and psychosis through my research and then finding this letter confirming my suspicions about Charley's behaviors being created by seizures provided a new incentive within me to share what we lived with others.

Along with psychosis there can be different types of delusions many of which Charley did not have. I do not believe a regular person has the ability to distinguish when another person is psychotic or has the ability to recognize when another person is delusional. When Charley was delusional he made irrational accusations or negative, untrue statements toward me or our children. I thought he was intentionally lying and was much more inclined to defend myself and our kids than deduce that he was delusional. How could an ordinary person know that? If you suspect the person you know who has epilepsy is psychotic and any delusional behaviors surface please do not take your suspicions for granted. Use the information I am providing to put the pieces together and get the person you love help. Make an appointment with their physician and explain the behavior to them. If possible make an appointment and first talk to the doctor without the delusional person present, otherwise you may unknowingly fuel their psychotic fire.

In the following chapters I describe different aspects of Charley's psychosis. Some of his behaviors were frightening, others funny and out of the norm. Though I had no medical proof for many years, I knew in my heart his erratic behavior was caused by seizures. His psychosis caused him to have irrational thought patterns and different needs than most people. He suffered with severe seizures many years before undergoing brain surgery and his case was rare. After his left temporal lobe was removed all the postictal behaviors caused by clusters of seizures vanished.

Charley suffered with a period of psychosis after surgery, but his behaviors were completely different than those caused by seizures. We will never know exactly why. For anyone dealing with a person who has epilepsy if any of these behaviors are familiar, speak to your treating physician about them. No one should have to suffer the way we did now that clusters of seizures and postictal psychosis are an indisputable and identifiable aspect of epilepsy.

Chapter 10
Explaining the Unexplainable: Understanding Delusions and Hallucinations

During the years I have been writing this book, tons of research regarding epilepsy and psychotic behavior has been ongoing. Many articles written by epilepsy specialists can be found on the internet that provide medical terms describing the behaviors of a psychotic person. These articles are written by physicians to provide research discoveries and information to other physicians. Doctors know the definitions of the medical terms. A regular person trying to survive living with epilepsy and the horrors that psychosis can create would have no clue what the terms mean much less have the ability to read the articles, decipher the medical terms and instantly realize they are dealing with psychosis. The articles I mention in the previous chapter use these terms to describe psychosis: delusions, depressive or manic psychosis, bizarre thoughts and behavior, auditory or visual hallucinations, abnormalities of content of thought, abnormalities of form of thought, mood changes, and aggressive behavior. In the following chapters I parallel Charley's behaviors to medical terms. There are behaviors Charley did not display that someone else who is suffering with psychosis might. This chapter is to help others who are researching and finding medical papers that describe psychotic behavior that includes delusions and hallucinations. It is frustrating to read research papers in the hopes of finding answers and walk away more confused than when you began.

On the occasions Charley had delusions I became madder than hell at him because everything he said was a lie. I thought he was just lying to get attention, but now I know he wasn't. What he was saying was real to him. Here are two examples:

We went to a store to purchase books. I put the books on the counter and as I paid the cashier Charley began visiting with her. He told the cashier that he (Charley) was going to college and that was why we were buying the books. He explained the classes he was taking and what he was majoring in and all kinds of absolute bull that was not even happening. I did not know he was delusional at that time, but I do now. When we got to the car I asked Charley why on earth he was telling such a big fib. He did not answer me and I honestly think he was trying to figure out what was going on as much as I.

Another example: We were each getting a hair cut at the same style salon. Charley was sitting several chairs down but I could hear him talking. The barber listened as Charley told him that his kidneys were shutting down and he was going to have to wear a bag to catch his urine for the rest of his life. We went to the same salon to have our hair cut for years so the stylists believed every word Charley said. Once again, I just thought he was lying but wondered then what the heck was going on. That is a pretty far stretch for a lie. Telling something like that to people we had known for years was extremely out of character for Charley. When I later asked him about the lie he just looked at me. He did not seem to register what I said. Again, I think he was trying to figure out what was going on. I now know Charley was having a somatic delusion which is the fixed, false belief that one's bodily function, sensation, or appearance is grossly abnormal (thinking your body is diseased in some way).

There are many different types of delusions. If you are involved with a person who has epilepsy and they speak what you think are lies maybe it is time to rethink the situation. A term often found while reading about psychosis and epilepsy in research papers is "**disorder of content of thought**" which simply means **a delusion or hallucination**.

Delusions

"A **delusion** is a belief that is clearly false and that indicates an **abnormality in the affected person's content of thought**. The false belief is not accounted for by the person's cultural or religious background or his or her level of intelligence. The key feature of a delusion is the degree to which the person is convinced that the belief is true. A person with a delusion will hold firmly to the belief regardless of evidence to the contrary. Delusions can be difficult to distinguish from overvalued ideas, which are unreasonable ideas that a person holds, but the affected person has at least some level of doubt as to its truthfulness. A person with a delusion is absolutely convinced that the delusion is real. Delusions are a symptom of either a medical, neurological, or mental disorder.

Delusions are categorized as either bizarre or non-bizarre and as either mood-congruent or mood-incongruent. A bizarre delusion is a delusion that is very strange and completely implausible for the person's culture; an example of a bizarre delusion would be that aliens have removed the affected person's brain. A non-bizarre delusion is one whose content is definitely mistaken, but is at least possible; an example may be that the affected person mistakenly believes that he or she is under constant police surveillance. A mood-congruent delusion is any delusion whose content is consistent with either a depressive or manic state; for example, a depressed person may believe that the world is ending, or a person in a manic state (a state in which the person feels compelled to take on new projects, has a lot of energy, and needs little sleep) believes that he or she has special talents or abilities, or is a famous person. A mood-incongruent delusion is any delusion whose content is not consistent with either a depressed or manic state or is mood-neutral. An example is a depressed person who believes that thoughts are being inserted into his or her mind from some outside force, person, or group of people, and these thoughts are not recognized as the person's own thoughts (called "thought insertion").

In addition to these categories, delusions are often categorized according to theme. Although delusions can have any theme, certain themes are more common. Some of the more common delusion themes are:

DELUSION OF CONTROL: This is a false belief that another person, group of people, or external force controls one's thoughts, feelings, impulses, or behavior. A person may describe, for instance, the experience that aliens actually make him or her move in certain ways and that the person affected has no control over the bodily movements. Thought broadcasting (the false belief that the affected person's thoughts are heard out loud), thought insertion, and thought withdrawal (the belief that an outside force, person, or group of people is removing or extracting a person's thoughts) are also examples of delusions of control.

NIHILISTIC DELUSION: A delusion whose theme centers on the nonexistence of self or parts of self, others, or the world. A person with this type of delusion may have the false belief that the world is ending.

DELUSIONAL JEALOUSY (or delusion of infidelity): A person with this delusion falsely believes that his or her spouse or lover is having an affair. This delusion stems from pathological jealousy and the person often gathers "evidence" and confronts the spouse about the nonexistent affair.

DELUSION OF GUILT OR SIN (or delusion of self-accusation): This is a false feeling of remorse or guilt of delusional intensity. A person may, for example, believe that he or she has committed some horrible crime and should be punished severely. Another example is a person who is convinced that he or she is responsible for some disaster (such as fire, flood, or earthquake) with which there can be no possible connection.

DELUSION OF MIND BEING READ: The false belief that other people can know one's thoughts. This is different from thought broadcasting in that the person does not believe that his or her thoughts are heard out loud.

DELUSION OF REFERENCE: The person falsely believes that insignificant remarks, events, or objects in one's environment have personal meaning or significance. For instance, a person may believe that he or she is receiving special messages from the news anchorperson on television. Usually the meaning assigned to these events is negative, but the "messages" can also have a grandiose quality.

ERETOMANIA: A delusion in which one believes that another person, usually someone of higher status, is in love with him or her. It is common for individuals with this type of delusion to attempt to contact the other person (through phone calls, letters, gifts, and sometimes stalking).

GRANDIOSE DELUSION: An individual exaggerates his or her sense of self-importance and is convinced that he or she has special powers, talents, or abilities. Sometimes, the individual may actually believe that he or she is a famous person (for example, a rock star or Christ). More commonly, a person with this delusion believes he or she has accomplished some great achievement for which they have not received sufficient recognition.

PERSECUTORY DELUSIONS: These are the most common type of delusions and involve the theme of being followed, harassed, cheated, poisoned or drugged, conspired against, spied on, attacked, or obstructed in the pursuit of goals. Sometimes the delusion is isolated and fragmented (such as the false belief that co-workers are harassing), but sometimes are well-organized belief systems involving a complex set of delusions ("systematized delusions"). A person with a set of persecutory delusions may be believe, for example, that he or she is being followed by government organizations because the "persecuted" person has been falsely identified as a spy. These systems of beliefs can be so broad and complex that they can explain everything that happens to the person.

RELIGIOUS DELUSION: Any delusion with a religious or spiritual content. These may be combined with other delusions, such as grandiose delusions (the belief that the affected person was chosen by God, for example), delusions of control or delusions of guilt. Beliefs that would be considered normal for an individual's religious or cultural background are not delusions.

SOMATIC DELUSION: A delusion whose content pertains to bodily functioning, bodily sensations, or physical appearance. Usually the false belief is that the body is somehow diseased, abnormal, or changed. An example of a somatic delusion would be a person who believes that his or her body is infested with parasites.

Delusions of control, nihilistic delusions, thought broadcasting, thought insertion, and thought withdrawal are usually considered bizarre delusions. Most persecutory, somatic, grandiose, and religious delusions, as well as most delusions of jealousy, delusions of mind being read, and delusions of guilt would be considered non-bizarre."

Delusions are a real part of epilepsy especially if a person is psychotic. If you are a caretaker or partner to someone you suspect is delusional get them help. Charley suffered with delusions and hallucinations of all types but I really did not know the extent of his misery with this disorder until recently. Research has helped me to identify some of his hallucinations. There were times that he was miserable because his mouth tasted like metal. This is called a gustatory hallucination. He also had occasions of smelling rancid odors that were not real. These are called olfactory hallucinations. Sometimes he thought other people were in the room with him when no one was. I know he heard voices, which is an auditory hallucination. He was admitted to a mental institution years ago for being suicidal. He told me he did not have any desire to kill himself but a voice was telling him that is what he needed to do. We never discussed the voice, mostly because I did not understand that the voice he heard was a separate being that he had no control over.

Hallucinations

"**AUDITORY HALLUCINATION**: The false perception of sound, music, noises, or voices. Hearing voices when there is no auditory stimulus is the most common type of auditory hallucination in mental disorders. The voice may be heard either inside or outside one's head and is generally considered more severe when coming from outside one's head. The voices may be male or female, recognized as the voice of someone familiar or not recognized as familiar, and may be critical or positive. In mental disorders such as schizophrenia, however, the content of what the voices say is usually unpleasant and negative. In schizophrenia, a common symptom is to hear voices conversing and/ or commenting. When someone hears voices conversing, they hear two or more voices speaking to each other (usually about the person who is hallucinating). In voices commenting, the person hears a voice making comments about his or her behavior or thoughts, typically in the third person (such as, "isn't he silly"). Sometimes the voices consist of hearing a "running commentary" on the person's behavior as it occurs ("she is showering"). Other times, the voices may tell the person to do something (commonly referred to as "command hallucinations").

GUSTATORY HALLUCINATION: A false perception of taste. Usually, the experience is unpleasant. For instance, an individual may complain of a persistent taste of metal. This type of hallucination is more commonly seen in some medical disorders (such as epilepsy) than in mental disorders.

OLFACTORY HALLUCINATION: A false perception of odor or smell. Typically, the experience is very unpleasant. For example, the person may smell decaying fish, dead bodies, or burning rubber. Sometimes, those experiencing olfactory hallucinations believe the odor emanates from them. Olfactory hallucinations are more typical of medical disorders than mental disorders.

SOMATIC/TACTILE HALLUCINATION: A false perception or sensation of touch or something happening in or on the body. A common tactile hallucination is feeling like something is crawling under or on the skin (also known as formication). Other examples include feeling electricity through one's body and feeling like someone is touching one's body but no one is there. Actual physical sensations stemming from medical disorders (perhaps not yet diagnosed) and hypochondriacal preoccupations with normal physical sensations, are not thought of as somatic hallucinations.

VISUAL HALLUCINATION: A false perception of sight. The content of the hallucination may be anything (such as shapes, colors, and flashes of light) but are typically people or human-like figures. For example, one may perceive a person standing before them when no one is."

Living with a person who is hallucinating or delusional is challenging. Not knowing the reasons for their behavior is a nightmare. Life should be more than a challenging nightmare for those now living with epilepsy. Charley and I managed to live a productive life in spite of having no answers to the nightmares that challenged us. Don't give up if you are seeking answers to questions that no one understands. More information is becoming available on a daily basis concerning epilepsy and psychotic behavior. Unfortunately, for people now living with epilepsy, those answers are hiding behind complicated medical terms written in confusing research papers. I hope my efforts answer some of the questions you are asking and guide you to seeking help with whatever unknown areas of epilepsy you are enduring.

Chapter 11

Living with the Bull: Recognizing Clusters of Seizures

Inside a fenced-in pasture is a huge bull owned by a rancher who is fairly new to cattle ownership. The rancher hired a professional consultant for advice on how to approach the bull in a way that might keep him from charging. The consultant (who studied bulls for years but has never been inside a fence with a bull) stands outside the fence and tells the rancher how to successfully approach the bull. The rancher, who knows the bull needs to become accustomed to sharing his pasture, steps inside the fence and closes the gate that the consultant has never entered. The consultant watches as the rancher slowly approaches the bull. The rancher keeps his pace as he observes the bull, knowing he will probably charge. Few times has the bull tolerated the presence of a human inside his fence. The observant consultant dutifully records the bull's actions for future reference.

The rancher questions his choice to spend hard-earned dollars on this consultant who is telling him to keep walking toward the bull. In spite of the consultant's advice the bull charges the rancher, who panics and runs. The consultant, still standing outside the fence, shouts, "Run, he is charging." as the rancher races toward the fence.

When the rancher opens the gate and narrowly escapes he shouts at the consultant, "I don't need you to tell me the bull is charging. I hired you to tell me how to approach him safely." At this moment the rancher realized the consultant had never entered the fence that contained the bull nor did he open the gate and help with quickly escaping the raging bull when the rancher was running for his life.

I give this analogy because Charley's nickname, aptly given by our sister-in-law Cheryl, was The Bull. There were many occasions he charged through life like a mad bull tearing up everything in his path because clusters of seizures were mentally pushing him so hard he could not slow down and control his physical actions.

Doctors are the consultants who medically treat people who have epilepsy and seizures. Most doctors, especially those who specialize in epilepsy, work hard to help their patients maintain a quality life. Unless a doctor has personally been the caretaker of a person who has seizures they will never step through the same gate, live inside the same pasture or run from the same raging bull that those who live with seizures are constantly trying to escape. Don't expect a consultant to share the pasture with you when you are trying to endure living with seizures. Doctors will never experience the panic, feel the fear, or know how to quickly open the gates and help with escaping the situations seizures create. Nearly one hundred percent of the time doctors cannot know seizures are occurring unless someone tells them, or the patient is placed under observation in a hospital to record their seizures.

Medical professionals who dedicate their life to studying and learning about epilepsy, seizures and brain illness are awesome. In the future they will find answers to seizures that we can only dream of having. When Charley and I began dealing with epilepsy brain surgery to eliminate seizures was unheard of. Now look at Charley's miraculous story; after twenty four years he beat epilepsy!!

What medical professionals are discovering about seizures is extremely important. The day will come when epilepsy is cured and no studies are needed to unlock secrets to seizure timing and duration. Sometime in the future no one will have seizures.

I lived many years observing Charley's illnesses slowly progress and his physical and mental abilities deteriorate. As seizures became more frequent he fought harder and harder to push them away. Charley was fighting for his sanity. Initially, only occasionally did he suffer with clusters of seizures that brought about a psychotic episode. As the years passed, and seizures occurred more often, the psychosis became frequent and odd behaviors emerged. Unlike now, I did not know then that Charley's irrational behaviors were a sign of clusters of seizures. We had no knowledge of clusters of seizures and I am sure many people today who are living in the same situation do not have a clue what they are.

When I began writing this book I looked for information about clusters of seizures on the internet. Dr. Diaz-Arrastia told us Charley was having clusters of seizures and that piqued my curiosity. I did not understand the doctor and thought he said cluster seizures. I initially thought that was another kind of seizure, like tonic-clonic or atonic. Eventually I realized Dr. Diaz-Arrastia had been referring to clusters of seizures which meant Charley was having multiple seizures. When I searched the internet using the terms cluster seizures or seizure clusters, for many years, the only information available concerned dogs having seizures.

I recently found a review, *Seizure Clustering*, written by Sheryl R. Haut M.D. She is an Associate Professor of Clinical Neurology and the Director of Adult Epilepsy at the Montefiore Medical Center, Albert Einstein College of Medicine. Her review about clusters of seizures is available online at sciencedirect.com.

In the review Dr. Haut states seizure clusters, flurries of seizures, repetitive, or serial seizures (different names for the same problem) are reported as occurring commonly in epilepsy. This is very important information that everyone who deals with seizures should know. A seizure cluster is a closely grouped series of seizures, or an increase over the patient's typical seizure frequency. Simple words. But what do those words mean to the people who actually live with epilepsy? Clusters of seizures medically represent a person having more seizures than usual. If a person normally has five seizures per day and seizure activity increases to ten a day are they having clusters of seizures? Or are the usual five seizures clusters of seizures to begin?

Dr. Haut goes on to say "there is no definitive clinical definition for a cluster or series of seizures. Some definitions used are; two to four seizures in less than 48 hours, three seizures within 24 hours, or two generalized tonic-clonic or three complex partial seizures within a four hour period." A lot of seizures might be referred to as a cluster of seizures. Before a person could be diagnosed with clusters of seizures they would most likely have to be admitted to an epilepsy unit and monitored. If that person had several seizures while under the constant monitoring of a medical team perhaps they would be diagnosed with clusters of seizures. Even then I wonder if those involved in this scenario would truly realize how severe and damaging clusters of seizures are.

Another aspect of epilepsy that Dr. Haut and many other experts are exploring is seizure timing. She states, "One of the unfortunate hallmarks of epilepsy is the unpredictability of seizures. The investigation of whether seizures are truly random events or events that follow identifiable patterns is not new."

There must be a relation between seizure occurrences and tons of other undiscovered factors. If someone unlocked the secrets to seizures and pinpointed an answer to when they will happen on an individual basis that would surely be a miracle. I learned to correlate the timing of some of Charley's seizures with identifiable behavior patterns. Millions of people living with seizures need answers that will make life more understandable. How many are living with clusters of seizures and have never heard of them or know the severe consequences if these seizures go unchecked?

Being diagnosed with clusters of seizures should be a startling wake up call that states very serious intervention must take place in order to get the seizures under control or eliminated. There is no going back when these seizures begin. You can only go forward and that is impossible if you have no idea how serious clusters of seizures are and will be in the future.

I read Dr. Haut's review with interest. We were unknowingly enduring clusters of seizures and Dr. Haut was studying them. I am elated the potential severity of constant seizures is recognized and being defined. Medical professionals are continually seeking answers to what we blindly managed to bear. An absolute conclusion being drawn as to the definition and exact timing of clusters of seizures will help with their management.

I witnessed two types of seizure activity with different variables. One type was definable because Charley's seizure's were seen and recognized. His visible seizures had names and distinct physical characteristics that allowed them to be studied and counted. Charley had episodes of non-stop tonic-clonic seizures that put him in the hospital many times. Those episodes absolutely were clusters of seizures.

The second type of seizure activity I saw was evident because of Charley's behaviors. Visible seizures did not always happen along with these behaviors but I knew seizures of some type were continually taking place. I did not have the word cluster for the seizures that were the creative force behind Charley's repetitive behaviors (that I now know were psychotic) but I knew he could not comprehend or remember his actions.

Seizure activity recognized through behavior is probably a known element of epilepsy by the medical community but I have found no references during research. I wonder how many people who are actually living within a world of epilepsy that is creating irrational behavior realize they could be dealing with clusters of seizures causing psychosis? That knowledge will create a more successful treatment of their epilepsy. Understanding behaviors that are caused by clusters of seizures creating postictal psychosis could place medical staff and patient's on a more even keel if everyone knew what to look for and how to deal with their findings. Epilepsy treatment needs to go beyond tunnel vision centered only on controlling visible seizures. Caretakers and family members with an active role in watching and studying the person who has seizures should pass behavioral information on to medical staff. If behaviors indicate psychosis is occurring, everyone should work together and learn how to take care of all the patient's needs. A person with epilepsy can also suffer with clusters of seizures that do not cause them to have irrational or psychotic behavior. In any event, if clusters of seizures are occurring medical intervention needs to take place.

When keeping an epilepsy diary be sure to record seizures and behaviors. Irrational, repetitive or unusual behaviors can happen before, between or after the occurrence of seizures. Clusters of seizures and psychotic behavior (especially patterns of behavior) could be more easily identified by taking a diary seriously.

Every doctor Charley consulted expected me to keep a diary of visible seizures and types. Not one of them ever inquired about repetitive irrational behavior. How can one thing have nothing to do with the other? Seizure behavior is as important as timing of seizures and their types. Patients and their families need to work with medical professionals interested in defining and counting seizures and also willing to study and comprehend behaviors that are a result of constant seizures. If you are not a member of epilepsy.com please go enroll on their site. There will be links on my website to their site for various helpful information. They have an online diary you can use for record keeping. When you go to the doctor the diary can be printed out.

Visible seizures with erratic behavior patterns between occurrences of those seizures is the first way I learned to identify the presence of clusters of seizures that were causing psychosis. I recognized that something was amiss and driving Charley's actions because he displayed the exact same behavior patterns days, months or years between episodes. I knew there was something repetitive happening within his brain creating the behavior and it was not chosen any more than he could choose to have seizures or always recognize them.

Sometimes Charley had seizures that were like a switch flipped on within his brain (instant misfiring neurons) then he recovered, and the "seizure switch" entirely switched off. Though he was physically ill from the seizure, he did not display psychosis before or afterwards. There were other times Charley did display psychotic behavior before, between, or after seizures. During events of psychosis it seemed Charley's "seizure switch" was halfway up and halfway down and misfiring current within his brain was constantly tormenting him. At that time he was definitely having clusters of seizures (sometimes for several days in a row). Charley may only have had one visible seizure within a week or month, which in medical terms (from my understanding) would not qualify as clusters of seizures, but the "seizure switch" never fully turning off resulted in him having constant (clusters, flurries, repetitive, serial) seizures that I recognized through his psychotic behavior (this behavior was psychosis caused by clusters of seizures but I did not know that at the time). The longer he had clusters of seizures the worse his behavior became.

Sometimes Charley's mind was charged and body continually on the go for days and nights on end. I knew some kind of seizures were, or had been, taking place simply by tuning into his behavior. Learn to recognize when a person's "seizure switch" is stuck between the on and off position and you can identify if constant currents are torturing their brain by studying their behavior. This is the way I recognized clusters of seizures were causing psychosis long before I knew there was a name for those seizures or understood the medical definition of what they were causing.

My experience with seizures does not use formulas and medical terminology that helps define seizure clustering as Dr. Haut's informative article does. Her review is full of knowledge from medical professionals who study and care for individuals who have epilepsy. Gathering, studying and basing conclusions concerning seizures on this type of information will definitely help with ministering to seizure patient's needs. The medical community will eventually define how often each type of seizure must occur before a person is clinically diagnosed as having clusters of seizures.

Charley's clusters of seizures did not always show physical attributes you would expect to see from a seizure. When he showed the slightest indication of a visible seizure warning I was immediately ready to physically brace him. If his behavior went awry, indicating a different outcome to his seizure activity, I mentally braced myself. If you are the caretaker or partner of a person who has epilepsy learn to be as prepared to spot behaviors that indicate seizures are, or have been, occurring as are you are to brace the person you love for a fall. The physical and behavioral aspects of seizures really are relative.

As an individual married to a person who had severe seizures I cared about understanding Charley's indescribably miserable behaviors that sporadically ruled our life. I had little knowledge about clusters of seizures during his lifetime and still, after seeking information, have learned clusters of seizures are a medical anomaly that is not yet defined.

In Charley's case the pattern I learned to identify was: the "seizure switch" remaining halfway on and halfway off for a period of several days causing electrical current to torment his brain, rule his actions and create psychotic behavior. Sometimes the psychotic behavior followed his having visible seizures and others not. The behavior always ended with a round of severe tonic-clonic seizures. To this day I do not know if Charley had seizures that I could not see (or did not see because I was working and not always with him) that caused his psychotic behavior before the tonic-clonic seizures occurred or if the psychotic behavior was caused by chemical imbalances (or a seizure switch being stuck) that precluded the seizures. Since I did not know what I was dealing with regarding clusters of seizures or postictal psychosis I did not make notes and correlate what type of seizure or frequency of seizures he had prior to episodes of extreme psychotic behavior. I did, in time, realize that the psychotic behavior stopped after tonic-clonic seizures occurred.

Knowing what behaviors to look for in the individual you love may help convince medical staff that clusters of seizures are occurring. My intent is to help others tie seizures and psychotic behavior together to create understanding. If you suspect the person you love is being tormented by clusters of seizures keep a diary of seizures and behaviors.

Now I know.

I could be a millionaire if I had a dime for every lesson looking back on Charley's epilepsy has taught me. No doctor, unless they live with someone who has seizures, is going to have a clue when behaviors indicate seizure activity. You cannot fault the medical community for that. It is the responsibility of caretakers and the person who has seizures to recognize irrational behavior and report such to their physician. Then medical staff must listen to the patients and/or their caretakers and try to control the seizure activity and behavior and whatever is causing both.

When Charley's mental being was completely pushed over the edge by constant seizures and he displayed psychotic behavior he never remembered his actions. Nor did he remember when he had visible seizures, but he should have kept a diary of his behaviors. When Charley's mental disposition did not reach far extremes he had the ability to weigh out situations. Many times he recognized irrational thoughts and actions and knew his entire being was out of character. He tried but could not get control of himself. Those times were many and Charley suffered greatly fully realizing he was gradually losing control of his mental existence. He asked for help from more than one doctor with the exact words, "I need help; my behavior is out of line." No one understood.

There may never be an exact clinical definition for clusters of seizures but there are four words that humanly define them - physical and mental torture. Consider clusters of seizures as countable and physical.

A severe seizure, such as a tonic-clonic is the result of a misfire within the brain that commands every single muscle in the body to operate simultaneously and are extremely exhausting. The physical toll on a body wracked with constant seizures can leave a person literally on the brink of death. I often wondered how Charley survived. His entire body became rigid for several minutes and sweat poured out of every pore on his skin during seizures. The strain resulted in horribly sore muscles when he was lucky and pulled muscles if not. Charley had no sense of security, knowing even a walk across the room might cause injuries if he fell. He was drained of energy from taking anti-seizure medications in high doses. When Charley had repetitive seizures he laid in bed and suffered because of an illness his mind did not understand that his body was forced to endure.

With no choice Charley and many other people are robbed of their independence by a physical force within their brains no one has found a way to control. They become dependent upon others to supply every need, the last thing anyone wants. They suffer with unexpected loss of bladder control, unexplained bumps, bruises, cuts, scrapes, pulled muscles, and haunting lapses in memory. If a person is having seizures that are within close enough proximity to each other to count them in order to try and classify them as clusters of seizures then you can aptly define those seizures, clusters or not, as physical and mental torture.

Doctors say that seizure clustering is lots of seizures or a person having more seizures than usual. The one problem I find with this conclusion is it seems to imply that everything important about seizures can be recognized. People living with epilepsy may not know clusters of seizures are occurring. We lived with seizures for more than twenty years before ever hearing the words seizure clustering. Even then, hearing the words did not tell us their meaning.

Defining seizure timing in order to identify clusters of seizures is important as well as teaching those who live with epilepsy and seizures how to recognize all seizure activity. A person falling because of daily seizures lives in a bad situation. Even worse are constant seizures that push someone beyond any level of sanity and cause them to be a danger to themselves or society. An insane individual driving down the highway whose actions are caused by continual seizures taking them into a world of psychosis is a much worse scenario than a person falling down within the confines of their home. Don't get me wrong, neither situation is good. We recognize the seizures of the person who falls yet very few people are familiar with irrational behaviors a constantly misfiring brain produces.

In reading Dr. Haut's review one thing stands out clearly. There is no absolute definition for clusters of seizures. Her work reveals that seizures are very complex and much about them is unknown. Because of medical professionals like Dr. Haut people who suffer with clusters of seizures will eventually be helped. In the meantime, during the next visit with your physician ask him or her if they are aware of clusters of seizures and postictal psychosis. Ask about any warning signs that indicate those seizures or behaviors may be occurring. Educate yourself, and always be on the lookout for repetitive physical seizures and take them seriously. Do not think having constant seizures is common like Charley and I did.

In retrospect I can identify changed behaviors of Charley's that gradually happened because clusters of seizures were tormenting him. His behaviors were not normal for him and cannot be used as an exact measurement against potential behaviors of other people. Someone else who has seizures may display odd behaviors that are nothing like Charley's but are abnormal for them and indicators of constant seizure activity.

The first sign of seizures taking over Charley's entire physical and mental being was repetitive psychotic behavior patterns which are explained in the next chapter. This psychotic behavior was uncommon initially happening sometimes months, and years, apart. Behavior patterns were always followed by a round of severe tonic-clonic seizures. After the seizures occurred and a recovery period passed Charley came back to being himself. He was sore, sick, tired and damaged but his aggressive intimidating behavior stopped, along with the seizure occurrences.

The next abnormal behavior that gradually infiltrated our life was insomnia. We both were sleep deprived for years. During most nights Charley could only sleep for a few minutes or hours at a time. His doctors prescribed medication but sleep always eluded him. During the first several years of our marriage Charley chose to watch television in bed before he went to sleep. As his insomnia worsened having the television on became a need and not a choice. Charley could not lie still and find any peace without the sound of the television overriding the constant roaring within his head. The light and sound from the television drove me nuts, so we compromised. He wore headphones while he watched television which kept me from hearing the sound. I slept with a pillow over my head to reduce the light.

Watching television was not a silly habit that Charley could change. Sleep came in short phases, an hour or two at the most, even with the television on. I learned not to turn the television off if he was sleeping with the headphones on because he was instantly awake. **It is not normal for a person to have a need for constant noise blaring in their ears in order to sleep.**

Clusters of seizures caused Charley to suffer from sleep deprivation. He hated wasting a day and saw himself as lazy if he took a nap. In time he forced himself to stay awake all day after having slept very little at night. This brought on two battles in his brain; fighting seizures and fighting sleep. It was horrible to witness Charley's gradual mental decline as he suffered with insomnia. He was totally exhausted every day blundering through life barely holding onto his sanity. **It is not normal to own a brain that never allows a body to rest.**

Throughout the first years of our marriage Charley was a well groomed man. In time continually fighting seizures caused him to lose his grip with reality and slowly slip into a loss of personal hygiene habits. Clusters of seizures robbed Charley of his self-awareness. Surviving life became such a struggle that personal hygiene was not something he was capable of. During bad episodes Charley did not bathe for days in a row unless I made him. He quit shaving and trimming his beard and brushed his teeth only when reminded but would not use toothpaste. He skipped washing his hair or rinsed it but stopped using shampoo and cream rinse.

Charley not being well groomed became a huge source of contention. I finally realized his mind should have been telling him to bathe but it was not functioning well enough to allow his body to feel the water or enjoy being clean. I tried in every way possible to help him stay connected to who he really was. I began trimming his beard, bathing him, shampooing his hair and shaving his face while he sat in the bathtub. I put toothpaste on his toothbrush and stood by while he brushed his teeth the way he did before becoming so sick.

I made sure that Charley's personal hygiene was attended to. This life became our normal because he was tormented by constant seizures. The thought never occurred to me that other women did not bathe their husbands or coach them through brushing their teeth. **It is not normal for a person to lose touch with lifelong personal hygiene habits.**

The year before Charley's surgery he was pushed beyond the levels of sanity by constantly fighting seizures. I picture these mental wars the same as a person grabbing a live electric wire and having the voltage running through their body yet using their mental capacities to make themselves stop feeling the shock. We jump away when shocked but Charley's short-circuit was within his brain and he could not let go of the current or avoid the shock. He trained himself to carry on and forced himself to not feel the shock of the currents.

Charley had many visible seizures that indicated he was suffering with clusters of seizures. The unseen mental war he fought . . . the continuous current . . . the motion within his brain of trying to let go of a voltage that was constantly shocking his brain, for Charley, was a second definition behind the term clusters of seizures. That battle created every type of psychosis, exhaustion, and a gradual loss of specific personality characteristics. **Clusters of seizures are scrambled brain signals that run a person, tire the body, confuse thought patterns, and create weird behavior.**

If you think the person you love may be suffering from clusters of seizures watch for an onset of behaviors that oppose their normal behaviors. **Something is wrong if a person changes from having perpetually good habits to indescribably bad ones.** If they are on the road to clusters of seizures ruling their life they will not be able to recognize those seizures for what they are or help themselves. **People do not consciously choose to change in negative ways.**

I lived inside the fence with The Bull and that was very difficult. Because of the deep love and commitment I felt toward my husband

I did not step out of the fence until God opened the gate and called Charley to heaven and made him whole again. Only then did I unwillingly escape his illnesses, twenty-six years after I walked into his pasture. I still miss my Charley.

When trying to survive within a pasture surrounded by hidden fences that are created by living with epilepsy the abnormal can slowly creep into your soul and become normal.

I look back so you can look forward;
And keep that from happening in your life

Chapter 12

Postictal Psychosis
and
Behavior Patterns

This chapter describes Charley's psychotic behaviors caused by clusters of seizures that coincide with medical definitions such as bizarre thoughts, violence, irritability and aggressiveness. Due to clusters of seizures Charley displayed repetitive behaviors months, or years between episodes. His behaviors following the same pattern were my clue that seizures were causing the insanity we endured. I have experience with one individual who had epilepsy and am writing about my observations and opinions which have not been confirmed by the medical community.

Imagine having an argument with someone in January and six months later that person repeating the statements and displaying the same physical moves during another argument. There were specific psychotic behavior patterns Charley displayed when clusters of seizures were tormenting his brain. I thought circumstances in life caused him to be irrational but situations were not the cause of Charley's behavior. His brain was having clusters of seizures and he would have displayed repetitive behavior because of this, regardless of life circumstances. He was not capable of memorizing his words or actions when suffering clusters of seizures. The only way he could repeat the behaviors months between events was for his brain to be misfiring exactly the same during each event.

Repetitive behavior was a symptom of Charley's misfiring neurons pushing his brain over the edge and creating psychosis. He displayed extreme frustration and/or agitation which always worked up to senseless unjustified anger. Charley could not mentally intervene with his anger and it grew until no rational words or apologies calmed him.

Before I describe Charley's behavior I want to visually establish the extent of his anger. The dictionary describes each degree of anger in these graduating terms: annoyance, anger, indignation, rage, fury, and wrath. Anger and annoyance are basic feelings we all can relate to. Annoyance is a feeling of irritation that is milder or more fleeting than anger. Compound the simple feelings of anger and annoyance and the anger graduates to resentment which is subdued anger caused by a sense of unfair treatment, and a powerlessness to remedy it. Indignation is anger based on a condemnation of something considered wrong or unfair. Add resentment and indignation together and the anger graduates to fury, an intense form of anger that suggests lack of control and potential to do violence. Mix together resentment, indignation, and fury and the anger graduates to rage: a violent anger that is the result of unstoppable fury. Visualize stirring the preceding types of anger into one pot with wrath (strong anger accompanied with overtones of a desire for revenge) and pour the mixture of all the angers into the soul of a person and you can see exactly how consumed with anger that Charley was.

Charley's psychotic behavior patterns began with mild anger but I knew by the empty look in his eyes nothing was going to calm him. Before I learned how to successfully deal with him if I tried to verbally calm him, a backlash of resentment kicked in and he would tell me how horrible I was with harsher words than anyone should ever hear. If I attempted to hug Charley and soothe his anger he shoved me away with seething anger and indignation. He was psychotic, his mind locked into rage, body in constant motion, and inner being determined to intimidate. Ignoring Charley made him furious and he shouted in my face to command my attention. During periods of Charley's psychosis he seemed to be repaying me for some horrible evil I had committed. I never discovered what he thought that evil was, and eventually I quit trying.

When these episodes occurred his anger built into rage, rage, rage; anger in unstoppable motion; intense, furious, loud, threatening. Raging anger in control of a person, pacing from room to room, shouting threats, slamming doors as he stomped outside and then slamming them again when he stomped back in. He was lost within anger, a raging maniac, uncontrollable, not able to comprehend his own words. Loud, hateful, demeaning words aimed at me and sometimes our innocent children. Cruel words meant to wound our hearts and push us to the point of confrontation. Charley paced, paced, paced as ugly words flowed out of his mouth blaming, blaming, blaming me for causing him to be mad. Furious, enraged, irate, seething, livid, anger beyond any expression of words and not one effort I made to calm Charley helped. The more I tried to appease him the more intense the anger and intimidation became. In Charley's case this behavior carried on (sometimes for days or weeks) during episodes of postictal, interictal, peri-ictal and whatever-ictal psychosis he had.

As Charley paced around the house he justified his actions by blaming others for creating his anger and did not understand anger as a chosen emotion. One sign of Charley's clusters of seizures creating psychosis was the inability to recognize or shut off his anger. (Medical terms: mood changes, violent, aggressive, delusional, bizarre thoughts and behavior).

Charley sometimes became furiously violent and destroyed our possessions. Many years ago Charley ripped all of our kitchen cabinet doors off of their hinges and threw them across the room. He had severe seizures the same night and the next day did not remember any of his violent actions. He built and hung new doors on the cabinets and cried as he apologized for committing such a horrendous act that he could not remember.

When Charley was psychotic many times he made a point of driving away angry. He drove away leaving dust flying and a trail of tire marks from peeling out in the car and then quickly returned . . . slamming on the vehicle's brakes and skidding to a stop directly on the same tire marks he had only moments before left behind. He slammed the car door when he exited and then came in the house and paced from room to room with his arms straight up in the air as if to force a release of anger out of the end of his fingertips. He repeatedly made the exact same statements trying to intimidate me and pick a fight (aggressive behavior). When I did not react he stood in doorway of the room I was in and unrelentingly stared at me.

Our children and I witnessed Charley display these repetitive behaviors for more than twenty years when clusters of seizures drove him into a world of psychosis. Sometimes months passed between episodes but the look in Charley's eyes, seething anger, and ugly words were always the same. I learned to not react or intervene. I could not help and any efforts I made to ease his frustration created confrontation. His behavior sometimes carried on all night. I tried to go to bed and encouraged him to do the same but his brain would not shut down.

During extreme psychotic episodes when I was lying in bed (trying to ignore him) Charley woke me up over and over, obsessively angry about situations that had occurred (or he imagined had happened). Sometimes he jerked the pillow out from under my head or jumped on the bed and landed with his knees straddling me. He marched around like an angry soldier keeping me awake by slamming doors and repeatedly turning the bedroom light on and off. Eventually I got out of bed and went to the living room. Exhaustion, frustration, fear and I sat alone and awake on the couch all night and said nothing in order to appease Charley's needs. I think he was scared and needed my company in spite of the fact that neither of us could halt his actions.

When Charley was psychotic I thought he was intentionally lying about situations that he described to pick a fight. Thirty years later I know he was having paranoid delusions and hallucinating. He believed the circumstances he described were real and his anger justified.

Charley's psychotic modes of rage and behaviors, months between episodes, were predictable step-by-step. I knew he was having seizures long before hearing the term clusters of seizures. Eventually I could predict his forthcoming actions 99% of the time. I knew when Charley was going to slam a door, come in the room, stare at me, get a glass of water and stare at me while he was drinking it, when he would go outside, and when he would leave. Charley tried to intimidate me when he was having these psychotic episodes. I refused to be intimidated by psychosis (I'm not claiming to be the smartest chick on the block).

Instances of psychosis are extremely irrational and sometimes dangerous. Learn to recognize psychotic behavior patterns and do not ignore them. I want to stress that Charley had seizures of one kind or the other on a weekly basis and almost daily when his psychosis ran rampant. His extreme psychotic behavior usually lasted about a week and sometimes longer and sometimes preceded tonic-clonic seizures.

That does not mean he had no other seizures prior to the days his psychotic behavior began. Sometimes he had seizures and others it seemed his seizure switch was stuck and his brain was tortured with a constant current that was not strong enough to produce a full-fledged seizure.

When Charley first started displaying psychotic behavior I thought he was the biggest jerk in the world. When psychotic he was an angry walking seizure and not a person that could possibly control his actions. It took a long time to put the pieces of the puzzle together and realize his behavior was caused by seizures. I learned to keep my cool but I was scared.

Sometimes when in a psychotic state Charley attempted to fix things but actually destroyed them. The battery cables on our car were loose and instead of getting a wrench and tightening them Charley pounded them with a hammer and broke the posts off the battery. He became physically violent during his psychotic episodes and threatened me, our home and family. He stated the exact same threats word for word even when the events were months apart. I learned to not feed into his behavior and watched his every move. I could say I loved or hated him and get the same angry, ugly reaction from him with either statement. I tried a million different things to calm and avert his behavior and not one of them worked. If the person you know displays psychosis do not feed into their behavior. Stay calm and try not to react in any way.

I can make a ton of suggestions of what not to do when dealing with a psychotic person but I cannot suggest exactly what to do. Each seizure situation is unique. Psychotic behavior is horrible. If Charley became psychotic when our grandchildren were visiting I took them home. Our children were not so lucky. I did not understand epilepsy and realize Charley's behavior was due to seizures.

If you know someone who has epilepsy and repetitive irrational behaviors occur and you know those behaviors are not normal please seek help. Talk to your treating physician and emphasize the severity of the situation. Don't doubt yourself or feel shameful of the circumstances and hide them like I did. Charley should have been on some type of medication for his irrational behavior for years. We explained his behavior to doctors but they did not understand and there was no information concerning epilepsy and psychosis available.

Charley could not remember his actions but did fully realize his behavior was out of line and pleaded for help. How can you explain psychosis when you do not know what it is? Who is going to believe you? Clusters of seizures causing psychosis comes from within the brain of a person who has seizures and is not caused by any circumstance other than living with an illness most people cannot comprehend.

Charley was arrested after an extreme violent outburst due to clusters of seizures. That forced me to find the help he needed. We began going to the University of Texas Southwestern Medical Center (in Dallas) to epilepsy specialists who actually knew about clusters of seizures causing psychosis. Receiving verbal confirmation from a neurologist that seizures were causing psychotic behavior was a great relief. I stuck by Charley in spite of the insanity because I knew he would never intentionally terrorize our family. I had no proof other than my own heart-felt conclusion that abnormal actions were normal for a person whose brain was torturing him because of epilepsy.

Recent medical research papers state that the longer a person has seizures the more likely they are to develop psychosis (generally symptoms will develop after ten to fifteen years). That should be the catalyst for everyone who has epilepsy (especially people who have tonic-clonic seizures) to try and eliminate their seizures through brain surgery if that is a viable option. We waited until Charley's seizures were completely out of control to seek brain surgery because we were afraid. **We should have been more afraid of the psychosis than the surgery** (you will see that statement written more than once in this book). Review medical research often, never give up on being seizure free and do not let the inability to define what is happening with your seizure situation prevent you from seeking answers.

We did not agree to brain surgery only because Charley was physically falling over from seizures. One of the most important reasons we agreed to the surgery is he was constantly having clusters of seizures and his psychosis never stopped. For more than a year before Charley's surgery psychotic behavior tormented the both of us twenty-four hours a day. I portrayed him as living in "loony land" on the initial paperwork I filled out when we went to the epilepsy clinic in

Dallas because he was extremely out of touch with reality. After his left temporal lobe was removed he never had another seizure or displayed the behavior patterns described in this chapter.

Chapter 13
Chronic Psychosis and Bizarre Behavior

This sentence is from *The Annals of General Psychiatry* concerning clusters of seizures causing postictal psychosis, "Chronic psychoses may develop from recurrent episodes or even a single episode (of postictal psychosis)." Those few words carry tons of meaning. Initially, in our life, Charley was psychotic occasionally. As time passed and more seizures occurred he developed chronic psychotic behavior patterns that slowly invaded his being even when clusters of seizures were not creating psychosis.

I have researched in an effort to see if any information is available that might help others who are living with epilepsy and psychosis to recognize behaviors that could confirm their suspicions about psychotic behavior. Had we known what was happening within Charley's brain due to clusters of seizures we would have gotten medical help sooner.

There was a huge gap between medical definitions that fit Charley's behavior and my layman's descriptions of his actions. For instance, the information I referenced concerning postictal psychosis symptoms contained descriptions such as bizarre thoughts and behaviors, delusions, abnormalities of content and form of thought, mood changes, and aggressive behavior. In the previous chapter I described instant mood changes and violent and aggressive behavior. This chapter describes some of Charley's bizarre behaviors that were not too extreme but were signs of chronic psychosis.

Caretakers of a person who has clusters of seizures need more than medical definitions to help correlate a person's bizarre behavior to psychosis. I knew what we were living with was not normal and also suspected Charley was psychotic. No information was available about his condition to guide me down the right path. It seemed a very harsh diagnosis (especially coming from me) to conclude my husband was psychotic. We endured many years living deep within a black hole where his undiagnosed psychosis pushed us. I suffered, knowing my husband was miserable and needed help in ways no one would understand. All I could do was protect him as I witnessed seizures slowly steal his mental being.

When living with a psychotic individual confirmation of their psychosis is very important. Describing daily behaviors Charley displayed due to psychosis creates another avenue of recognition. His behavior was not always extreme but it did follow a pattern of abnormality. Charley was a unique individual in all aspects and his behaviors will not exactly match those of any other psychotic person. Charley's bizarre explanations regarding his behavior made me doubt myself and delayed my finding him help. Do not doubt yourself if you are witnessing psychotic behaviors, even if you are not sure your suspicions are correct. Distance yourself from the actions and be observant and you will know if a mind is being tormented by seizures.

As someone who lived with a psychotic person for many years I can provide good examples of psychotic behaviors. Charley's daily psychotic behaviors often exposed themselves as repeated personality traits that could be embarrassing, irritating and sometimes very funny but were basically harmless. Recognizing these traits as abnormal and unchangeable taught me to understand him and accurately predict his actions and reactions. I learned through his psychotic behaviors where we could and could not go in public, what he could manage and protected him from uncomfortable situations.

I was not perfect and it was not easy to live with Charley's psychosis. I constantly worked on learning to accept these traits as part of his personality. Everyone who knew us will tell you Charley irritated me half to death a lot of the time. In most marriages a couple can discuss bothersome personality imperfections and strive to be more pleasing to their spouse. Charley's psychotic personality traits were nothing that he could discuss or improve. He laughed and laughed when he could manage to irritate me to the point that I teasingly put my hands around his neck, pretended to choke him, and announced it was time for him to die and I intended to see to it that he did.

Had I not observed and sometimes grudgingly learned to accept

Charley's psychosis our marriage would not have endured. He knew my imperfections very well too and dealt more than fairly with my quirks, especially for a person with so many problems.

To learn Charley's behaviors I had to be observant. The only way to observe the behavior of another person is to shut up and allow them to completely finish, without interruption, whatever action they are taking or words they are stating. Before I accepted Charley's personality I had a tendency to correct him in the middle of whatever he was saying or doing when he was extreme. One day as I was correcting him I angrily said, "You do the same thing every time."

I was looking Charley straight in the eyes when I said those words. Something about the way he looked back at me made my words ricochet off of him and hit me straight in the heart. I could not speak and had to sit down. I sat with my elbows on my knees, fingers entwined in my hair, looking down toward my feet as I held my head in my hands. I was no longer correcting Charley or attempting to direct his behavior. I became engrossed in trying to remember a word I learned in college. After a few minutes of using every ounce of my brain power I recalled the word that was immediately so important: epiphany

My epiphany brought tears to my eyes and a message to my soul. I heard God telling me to listen as He was speaking directly to my heart. I get the chills writing about that moment. I heard the Lord speaking but was not happy with the message. "Listen to your words," the Lord whispered to my soul, "he does the same thing every time." Once again the lesson had to be learned that I could change and my husband could not.

I told Charley I was sorry for correcting him. He happily accepted my apology and, I am sure, thought no more of the incident but I did. The words, "he does the same thing every time" echoed throughout my soul. From that moment I worked to not over-correct Charley though I was not perfect. I also tried to see the humor in his psychotic traits rather than allowing my inability to control his behavior create unnecessary negativity in our life.

Charley walked on a plane about ten feet above others. His psychosis pushed him up there. He came down often, loved on people and tried to interact normally. Try as he may a lot of his interaction within the normal plane of life tended to be inappropriate, irritating and extreme. He did not always comprehend what he did wrong but recognized when others knew his actions were abnormal. He then mentally returned to his own plane of existence. Charley saw and experienced life in a different manner than others. Sometimes he was halfway between the two planes (normal and psychotic) and life was semi-normal. It never paid for me to grab onto Charley's feet and try to pull him down from his level of existence. The times I did try to force him down were when I was desperate to be understood. Charley did try but never completely comprehended most of my feelings. Even on days he did grasp my needs my requests were not within his ability to mentally reach by the next day. He had returned to his unique level of existence.

When Charley came down and tried to walk on the normal plane he experienced more problems with psychosis. He could disguise his chronic psychosis and fool everyone walking ten feet above them. Charley did not understand and could not grasp the all-encompassing rules in life that most people follow. Some of his actions and reactions were quite funny, others very frightening and dangerous.

When people were around Charley he knew they were there physically. He saw bodies, touched skin, and cherished being hugged. Nothing pleased him more than physical contact with another human being. Sharing the energy of others through touch helped Charley stay focused and not drift into the seclusion psychosis causes. From the inside looking out Charley was a very loving man who relished touch and affection. From the outside looking in he often seemed needy, attention starved, and overly aggressive.

A good way to picture the existence of someone who is psychotic is to imagine looking up and seeing the bottom of their shoes above you. They mentally walk at a faster pace than others and live on a different plane. Living with a psychotic person is exasperating but not impossible. Some episodes of psychotic behavior are more intense than others. I thought of Charley's psychosis as being present like a dog resting under a bush waiting for the delivery man. It may not be agitated enough to show itself and bite someone or may come out and only want to be petted but psychosis was always a mental part of my husband.

Being psychotic should not be a source of shame. It is

counterproductive to society to hide the personality factors that psychosis creates. No matter the cause of psychosis the psychotic person needs to be understood, loved and accepted. Charley used to tell me he had no problem talking to himself but it did tend to bother him when he did not know who was answering!

Charley's chronic psychotic behaviors were mostly mild, sometimes moderately extreme but overall harmless. One personality trait of Charley's psychosis was an intimidating manner. He did not have the ability to rationalize anything that upset him. Charley immediately started intimidating others if he felt unfairly treated. He spoke irrational words that revealed thoughts that were different than most peoples would be in upsetting situations. For example, Charley went to the bank to find out why our account balance was not matching the statement. He became agitated because he did not understand what the teller was explaining and threatened to follow her home and burn her house down. He never would have followed through on such a threat and admitted the teller was not rude but those threatening words escaped him. Confusion created inappropriate verbalization.

Another example: Charley was stopped by the police for speeding. I doubt many people can say they are thrilled to get a speeding ticket. Charley's thoughts were probably the same as most peoples are when stopped by the police but he spoke the words to the police officer we all know should not be said. The policeman told Charley to calm down or he was going to jail. He was intimidating with his manner, started laughing and told the policeman to calm his own self down. People who are drunk on the television show "Cops" make an ass of themselves by trying to intimidate with words. That is exactly how psychosis affected Charley, except he was perfectly sober. If Charley had a thought he said it, good or bad, nice or nasty, appropriate or inappropriate. He never backed down and was not afraid of any threat.

Another personality trait of Charley's psychosis was withdrawal within a crowd. He became agitated by the crowd's energy but literally did not see people. We went Christmas shopping at a mall the first time I recognized Charley's psychotic withdrawal within a crowd. We discussed our plans to shop individually and meet at a designated area within the next hour. We were excited at the prospect of having enough money to actually buy each other gifts.

We were surrounded in the mall by noisy crowds and the quick pace of herds of people. As we made our way through the crowd I could sense Charley's demeanor changing. He became combative and made rude remarks to people walking close to him. I suggested we leave and Charley became very angry. We crossed a line at that moment. I had no name for Charley's behavior but did recognize his withdrawal and inability recognize his behavior. My trying to accommodate him by offering what a normal person would need in a situation they were uncomfortable in made him angry.

We continued through the crowd and I designated a spot for us to meet when our shopping was done. Charley was very agitated and asked me, "What the hell are were doing at the mall?" I was dumbfounded and reminded him that we were Christmas shopping. I brushed off his weirdness and told him we would meet in an hour. I turned and walked maybe one hundred steps away and Charley loudly yelled, "Lola." He shouted at me because he was frightened, surrounded by the energy of a crowd and unable to see the source of the energy. He cried out for me to connect with a familiar energy.

Hundreds of people stopped and looked at Charley. I froze in place and slowly turned around. At that moment I realized he was standing within a crowd of people and did not see them. The unfamiliar atmosphere pulled Charley down from his level of existence and brought his psychosis to the surface. He was desperately trying to escape the insanity that was churning within his mind.

I walked to Charley, took his shaking hand and steered him through the crowd and to our vehicle as if he were blind. He thought I was angry. I was not angry but I don't exactly know what I was. The reality that something was wrong was undeniable. I made a mental list of all the activities we needed to avoid because I knew it would be best not to take Charley into another crowd. I went to the mall with my husband and came home with an agitated stranger. Somehow, in his mind, I had embarrassed him by exiting the mall. He did not remember screaming my name. After that I tried to avoid taking Charley to crowded places.

Another bizarre behavior of Charley's was striving to be the center of attention. Both of our son's played sports so we could not always avoid being in a crowd. Charley knew other people were in the bleachers but he did not care about their reactions to his overzealous behavior. He yelled "Kill the zebra!" at the top of his voice if he felt the referee made an unfair call. I wanted to wear a sack over my head. Charley shouted louder and louder and if I ask him to be quiet he told me to let him have fun. I could not sit beside him without wanting to kill myself so I sat a few seats away and left him alone as he yelled, whistled, and drew attention to himself. There was no stopping Charley's attention-seeking behavior.

We went to visit my cousin, Tom, and his wife, Sheila, in Oklahoma City. Tom took us to a movie rental store. Charley noticed a picture on one of the cowboy movies of a woman riding a horse. In front of a very prim and proper woman who was also shopping Charley very loudly said, "Tom, did you hear about the woman sheriff?" I froze. I had heard this joke six million times since we married. I nicely told Charley to hush but he wasn't about to until he loudly delivered the punch line, "She had a big posse." Tom laughed at my being mortified as much as he laughed at the joke.

Our friends said I spoiled Charley too much and that was why he had to be the center of attention. I did, but the constant need to be the center of attention was part of his psychotic inner being and had nothing to do with the external circumstances in his life.

When our daughter, Kate, was eleven years old and our sons, Chaeton and Alan, eight years old our family went on a camping trip to our favorite lake on the top of a secluded mountain in New Mexico. The lake is small, covering about four hundred acres when full. Camp sites are visible from across the lake but usually the campers can't be seen. The lake has a very serene and quiet atmosphere. Conversations spoken in a normal tone can easily be heard across the lake.

We had borrowed my dad's small boat that has a gas motor. After setting up camp the kids and I drove Charley and the boat to the dock for a grand launching. Older people had their campers parked near the boat dock because it is close to the lake's entrance. The mountain is very rocky and the "boat dock campers" apparently don't want to risk their vehicle's tires by driving any further than necessary to camp.

There were several older men fishing at the boat dock when we launched the boat, with Charley aboard, onto the lake. My dad had shown Charley how to start the boat motor but he apparently forgot the instructions. Charley pulled the rope like a madman and the motor sputtered. Kate, Chaeton, Alan and I stood on the boat ramp and watched as he repeatedly tried to start the motor. Charley pulled the rope and then let loose with a very loud string of curse words, "Lola, How in the hell do you start this *&^%$# boat motor?"

I answered him in a normal tone "Charley, turn on the gas."

He pulled the rope again, cursed the motor, and hollered, "What in the hell is wrong with this piece of #$%@ motor?"

I answered, "Charley, turn on the gas."

After a few minutes of Charley yelling every curse word in the book at the top of his voice and the sound of the boat's motor sputtering the kids and I had quite a crowd of elderly people standing around us. We all quietly observed Charley yanking on the motor's rope and loudly cursing as I calmly kept repeating, "Turn on the gas."

Charley was within his own world and did not hear me telling him to turn on the gas or see the crowd of spectators his goofy behavior had drawn. In front of this crowd Charley stopped pulling on the motor's rope, leaned over to the right, lifted his left butt cheek off of the boat seat and let loose with the biggest, longest, loudest fart I have ever heard in my entire life. Without a word spoken between us Kate, Alan, Chaeton and I turned around and started walking toward our vehicle. After a few steps I said to the kids, "Sounds like he got the gas turned on to me."

"Yep," the boys and Kate said in unison.

We left Charley drifting in the boat, climbed into our vehicle, and drove back to camp. Part of me was giggling; the other part was thinking what a handy time that would have been for Charley to drown. In a little while we heard the boat motor start and Charley came putting up to shore happy as he could be in spite of the large blisters on his fingers from madly pulling the rope. I asked Charley if he had enjoyed farting for everyone on the lake and he looked at me like I had lost my mind. He never did remember letting that fart and I never did forget because it was one of the funniest things the goober ever did.

Thousands of people let farts when they shouldn't and that does not mean they are psychotic. But, if those people let farts in front of a crowd that their inappropriate behavior has created and they have no clue they have drawn a crowd to within twenty yards of them then you could be dealing with a person who is psychotic. And, if the person has no memory of their inappropriate deeds within a few minutes of having committed them, you could be dealing with psychosis.

Two aspects of living with a psychotic individual have to be accepted. They may do or say things in front of anyone that will shock and embarrass you and whoever else is around. When Charley's actions were inappropriate I was stunned and could not believe what he had done. I learned to tell myself it is done and tried not to overcorrect. I did overcorrect but consciously tried not to. The second part of living with psychosis is understanding, and believing, the psychotic person cannot remember one whit of what they did. It is fruitless to try and encourage someone to change their behavior when they cannot remember their actions.

In essence at the same time you are saying to yourself, "I cannot believe what he/she did" you also have to say to yourself, "I have to believe he/she does not know what they did." Our society has a gut instinct to correct inappropriate behavior and we refuse to believe that a person could do something and not remember. Some chronic psychosis situations are funny, others humiliating and many are sad. Enjoy the humor and do not dwell on circumstances that are beyond your control.

Another aspect of Charley's chronic psychosis was being unreasonably uncomfortable with death. Charley thought he was never going to die and did not like being reminded that everyone will. This is an example of a grandiose delusion caused by psychosis. This type of delusion is a belief that is completely false and indicates an abnormality in the affected person's content of thought. The key feature of a delusion is the degree to which the person is convinced that the belief is true. It is hard to put these clues about psychosis together. I thought Charley was kidding when he said he was never going to die but I now understand he wasn't. He argued with me for hours once because he thought it was against the law to show a dead body on television. It was unfathomable to him that showing a dead body on television would not be unlawful. After attending funeral services Charley always looked at me with sad eyes and said he did not want to see the body and I always reassured him that it was fine to not want to look at a dead person. When other people were walking toward the casket to see the body for the last time we snuck out of the building. Death was an obstacle Charley's mind could not overcome. He did not process any thoughts about death correctly. Death pulled Charley down from his plane of existence very quickly because it was too frightening for his mind to do anything but deny. After attending funerals Charley always had seizures due to the emotional upset.

Another sign of Charley's chronic psychosis was not processing daily chores in a step-by-step manner. This behavior was one indicator of what is medically termed absence of the form of thought (another unexplained medical term used in research papers as an indicator of psychosis). Disturbances in the form of thought are disturbances in the logical processing of thought, or more simply, disturbances in the logical connection between ideas. The following paragraphs give examples of Charley's inability to logically connect ideas.

Charley mowed the lawn but never picked up the stuff in the yard before mowing. He mowed over or around everything that was in his path. Rather than pick up a big piece of paper before mowing he ran over it and created thousands of little pieces. He did not pick up rocks that had surfaced since the last mowing. He ran over them and damaged the mower blades. It did no good for me to ask Charley to pick up the stuff on the lawn before mowing. I was left with the choice to clean the lawn before he mowed, mow the lawn myself, or clean up the millions of little pieces of stuff he ran over and destroyed.

Another of Charley's bizarre behaviors was disregarding his own safety. We have a weed eater on wheels called a D.R. Trimmer mower and goggles must be worn for eye protection when using this tool. Charley refused to wear goggles and on two different occasions objects flew into his eye causing serious injury. I took over using this tool because it was beyond his capacity to take safety precautions even after being seriously injured. Charley refused to wear gloves when he worked with long sheets of sharp metal building portable buildings. He had to have stitches in his hands because of severe cuts, but still refused to wear gloves and protect his hands.

When Charley was outside he threw trash on the ground. When he emptied a bottle of water the bottle went on the ground. Sometimes he picked the trash up but most times not. In a vehicle Charley threw trash on the floorboard. No requests ever changed these behaviors. In our home he threw trash in the garbage but when he was outside trash went on the ground.

Charley did not check the oil or maintain our vehicles. He left the plug out of the oil pan and poured all the new oil through the motor and into a huge puddle on the ground the one time he tried. If he changed a flat tire I had to make sure all the lug nuts were tight or we might have a tire passing us on the highway. Charley's inability to fully and safely complete tasks is an example of a disturbance in the connection of logical ideas.

When Charley cooked food the fire was always turned on high. Smoke poured off the stove but he never turned the fire down unless I made him. Often the food was burned to a crisp but he never complained about the flavor.

Charley's chronic psychosis caused his mind to be stuck in fast gear and I believe that is why he could not logically connect ideas (no logical processing or ability to logically connect ideas). He did not have first, second, and third gear most people's minds use as they begin to accomplish tasks. Before mowing the yard first gear would be picking up stuff, second gear checking the oil in the mower and making sure the mower is in working order and third gear start mowing. Charley's brain was not able to stop and accurately process the steps necessary to begin tasks. If the yard needed mowing he mowed the yard and that was the end of the story.

There were many clues to Charley's psychosis had I known. Along with other characteristics of seizures it took years to understand their significance. One difficult aspect of living with psychotic behavior is accepting it as unchangeable. You can drive the psychotic person crazy by constantly demanding and expecting change and drive yourself insane with the disappointment of unfulfilled expectations.

Some of the defining factors of Charley's chronic psychotic behavior were his inability to recognize his actions as abnormal and the impossibility to change. If you live with a person who is chronically psychotic life will be much easier when the reasons for their behaviors are recognized and accepted. No amount of nagging is going to change the fact that their thoughts do not process correctly. Try to teach yourself to have repeated positive reactions to their repeated goofy actions.

The ability to cope, live with and enjoy a psychotic person depends upon two factors. The first is how much are you willing to give in order to deal with the psychosis? The second is how much are you willing to take in order to live with the psychosis.? The give and take of living with a psychotic person is a balancing act upon a fine line that is very hard not to fall off of once in a while.

Many times when I was impatient or having trouble dealing with Charley's bizarre behavior I lost my balance and fell off my fine line. Often it was my very own psychotic husband picking me up, wiping away my tears, hugging me, brushing me off, and telling me everything was going to be all right. And it was, wasn't it Charley? It was all right.

Chapter 14

Charley and Cheryl: Sparring Partners

Every family has one person that hardly anyone understands. That person is outspoken, tends to overstate their opinions, and frequently pisses off everyone. Their actions are often extreme and opinions are not what anyone wants to hear. This person's scorn is avoided at all costs but their love is treasured and valued because it is not false. This person is incapable of pretending regardless of the situation. They are honest whether praising another or blessing them out. Their love shines and warms like the sun and wrath chills to the very bone. Their friendship honors you because it is forever and true. But look out for that wrath!

In my family the person I am describing is my brother David's wife. Her name is Cheryl. I call her the volcano because she verbally erupts like a volcano when aggravated. No quicker than a thought enters her mind than that thought is verbally spewing out of her mouth. Many times I have seen Cheryl literally run when encountering an idiotic person because her verbal gate is broken. She darts away rather than spew her thoughts in front of a stranger who has no idea a verbal volcano is on the brink of erupting within their midst. Cheryl has tried to learn to whisper when necessary but whispering does not happen often. Usually Cheryl is loud and her verbal thought eruptions can be heard by everyone within a city block. I think she is hilarious . . . now . . . I used to be scared to death of her but now I totally understand her. I cannot help but hug her after a volcanic verbal eruption. Cheryl now fills an empty spot in my heart that Charley once fully occupied.

Charley did not make a good impression when he first met Cheryl. They only tolerated each other. Cheryl reminded Charley what an ass he was when they first met and did not mind telling him she did not think he had changed. Charley's response was, "there is no reason to change who I am in order to please an old bag like you." And that is how their relationship rocked along for years.

In 1996 David and Cheryl were sinking financially. Charley and I moved within close proximity of them. We spent a lot of time helping get their restaurant reopened after a temporary closing and remodeling. Charley worked hard and donated several months of his time, money and carpentry experience. Cheryl did not change her mind about Charley being an ass but she did tell him he was a "big-hearted ass" after he helped get their business reopened.

After opening the restaurant David immediately began drawing plans for the house Charley had always wanted to build. The tables turned, David and Cheryl spent countless weeks, hours and money helping Charley and I accomplish his life's dream of building a two-story house. David always said he had less knowledge in his entire body about carpentry than Charley had in his little finger. Though Charley's carpentry experience was immense his thoughts were scattered and follow-through poor due to his seizure condition. David once said that our house would have looked like the slanted room at the fair had he not continually monitored Charley's work. The statement was true because Charley's brain did not process thoughts correctly and not because he was lacking in knowledge.

David and Cheryl's time is very limited due to being business owners. Charley and I worked alone day after day building our house. Every evening after working all day at the restaurant David and Cheryl drove to our construction project. David was diligent to check our work and make sure his home design was being built correctly and would come to life in time. Charley never could have blueprinted the house plans. He valued the blueprints David drew but resented being told how to build a structure by someone with less carpentry experience.

David was on short time and trying to get Charley to follow the house plans. When David was giving Charley precise instructions rather than listen and apply the needed instructions he argued. Then Cheryl spoke. It did not take much of Charley arguing with David to blow the volcano. Cheryl was tired and frazzled and beyond caring if Charley's pride was wounded. She yelled and told him if he would shut the hell up and listen his house would be built twice as quickly. Cheryl told Charley the experience he had as a carpenter did not mean anything if our house ended up falling over because he refused to build the house correctly. Charley swelled up and loudly stated he knew how to build a house without anyone's help. Cheryl told him he might know how to build a house without anyone's help but she sure as hell would not walk in the door for fear the entire structure might fall on her head. Then Charley ended the argument with, "Good, I don't want your ass in my house anyway."

Very seldom did Cheryl get angry at Charley during our construction days but he got angry at her. There was not much he could do about his aggravation because he knew she was right. Cheryl was not backing down or apologizing for her statements. The more lip Charley gave her the more she happily gave in return.

An essential friendship was born between Charley and Cheryl. They became sparring partners. David loved to see Charley walking in the door. He gladly took the hot seat and gave David a break from Cheryl's spewing volcano eruptions. When Charley's moods were out of line I did not always wait for Cheryl to visit. He griped and grumbled and nit-picked at me until I could not stand to hear another word out of his mouth so we got in the car and went to where Cheryl was so they could have a good fight. If I told Charley he had life pretty good in spite of his illness he became very angry. Cheryl told Charley he was the most spoiled man in the universe and the fight was on. Charley told Cheryl (who worked on her feet at least 12 hours a day every day) the only reason she thought he was spoiled was because she was LAZY! Then Cheryl spewed at Charley and told him the reason he thought she was lazy was because he was a complete IDIOT that would not know reality if it hit him square in the face. Then Charley told Cheryl if she wanted to see an idiot to go look in the mirror. This banter went on all day.

There were times Charley picked at Cheryl and eventually made her so mad she got in his face and screamed at the top of her lungs at him. When Charley actually made Cheryl mad enough to scream at him his day was completely, totally, one hundred percent made. Nothing put Charley in a better mood than to make Cheryl mad enough to scream in his face. He giggled the rest of the day. "Made the old bag mad." Charley said as he snickered his way through the day.

But Cheryl always got her revenge. Sometimes she picked at Charley and eventually said enough that he would pucker up and pout. For the rest of the day Charley silently pouted, sent dirty looks at Cheryl and refused to say a word to her. When Cheryl actually made Charley mad enough to pout her day was completely, totally, one hundred percent made. Nothing put Cheryl in a better mood than to make Charley pout. "Made the jackass pout." she said between giggles, "He thinks he is getting back at me but I am glad he finally shut the hell up."

There were times when they fought that every person within range of them cleared the room, including David and I. They got into shouting matches no one wanted to witness. We figured they were each too mean to kill the other so we let them go at it and enjoyed our relief from the hot seat.

I absolutely know Charley having this crazy relationship with Cheryl was one of the healthiest aspects of his life. I also know that Charley loved Cheryl with a love much deeper than most people have the ability to feel because she was honest and her love was not false. Cheryl's love warmed Charley like the rays of the sun and her friendship honored him until the day he died.

I used to try and keep them away from each other because their verbal wars made everyone uncomfortable. David pointed out to me how much fun the two of them had running each other down and expressing everything that happened to be a thought. Sharing broken verbal gates made each of their worlds a happier place in the most indefinable way.

A psychotic person has many unusual needs. One need Charley had that Cheryl fulfilled was to be himself and be allowed to fight. He could not be himself with me because he hurt my feelings and I did not want to spar and certainly could not scream in his face.

If you are lucky there is one person like Cheryl in every family. Get to know them instead of being intimidated by their honesty and there is no truer friend. Even when pouting Charley's spirits were always lifted after seeing Cheryl. He knew whatever verbal punch she had thrown was well deserved. He always looked forward to his next opportunity to "give that old bag hell."

I have always had Charley and Cheryl stories to tell but my favorite happened a few years ago. David bought a building that needed remodeling in order to move his restaurant into a facility with a banquet room and new kitchen. Charley helped with this construction project. One afternoon we were working and Cheryl drove up and parked.

Charley looked over in her direction then said, "I bet she is here to tell me how yellow my teeth are."

What the hell? Of all things I anticipated him saying one of them was not that Cheryl had driven to where we were working to tell Charley how yellow his teeth were. I dumbly stared a hole through him. I thought he must have misspoken his words or was going to soon have a seizure. "He must be scrambled." I said to myself, but after several moments I could not say a word. About the time I decided my best bet would be to completely ignore him Cheryl came storming into the building. It was a sure thing Charley had made her mad, but he was pouting so we had a tie in the sparring match. Apparently neither of them had declared themselves the winner and walked away giggling from their latest verbal war.

Cheryl marched past Charley and asked me if he told me what happened. "Nope." I said as I shook my head.

Then she said, "I was bringing him back after cooking him lunch. He started kicking the stuff on the floor of my car telling me I am lazy because my car is not perfectly clean. I fixed him lunch, came and got him, fed him, and drove him back and that is all he can say." (No matter how tired or busy Cheryl was she always made sure Charley was fed because of his seizures. She was convinced if I fed him right he would not be sick(that is the kind of stuff you hear from the one person).

Then Charley innocently pipes in, "Well, the car is messy and I told her she needs to clean the damn thing." Then he said, "She pulled the car over."

He looked at me like I was going to defend him. I could not guess what was coming. Cheryl was steaming (when she gets really mad her green eyes practically pop out of her head and they were popping big time).

She said, "You're damn right I pulled the car over. I was going to throw his ass out on the street. I asked him if he wanted me to knock those damn yellow teeth down his throat – and I still might do it." She stormed away, got back in her car, slammed the door and drove away. I honestly do not know how long Charley pouted or how long Cheryl was mad. I do know that was the funniest sparring event they ever had. Neither of them walked away giggling, but David and I did. It was hilarious to see each of them mad at the same time.

David and Cheryl brought an ice cold watermelon to our house every Sunday after Charley's brain surgery. That was one of his favorite foods. Cheryl lovingly teased with Charley and encouraged him to get back to normal (whatever the hell that meant Charley would say). The visit always ended with Cheryl giving "the old fart" a hug as she told him to hurry and get well so they could fight again.

When Charley healed enough to spout off at Cheryl they stepped comfortably back into their verbal boxing ring.

Cheryl was one of the greatest gifts God ever gave to Charley. He enjoyed their verbal wars tremendously. After Charley died, at his life celebration, Cheryl sweetly sang a song called The Anchor Holds in tribute to her sparring partner. Everyone was very moved.

David was the speaker at Charley's life celebration, who better? When Cheryl finish singing David gave her time to wipe the tears no one was supposed to see from her eyes, and said, "If Charley were alive and here right now he would look at Cheryl and say thank you, you old hag." You can surely bet Charley would have done just that.

Our Journey
to
and
Through
Brain Surgery

Chapter 15
Our Point of No Return

The last episode of postictal psychosis caused by clusters of seizures pushing Charley over the edge that occurred in our household was caused by a progression of bad choices. The situation that led up to this event did not happen overnight and involved Charley, me and our daughter Katie.

Katie was going through a divorce. She and her two children moved into a rent house in a small town near where we live. Kate was also paying payments on a house she owned that we spent months repairing and were trying to help her sell. She could not make ends meet. I told her to move in with us. I knew the situation would be hard on Charley but there really was no other option. In order to get Kate out of debt and help with a fresh start we invested a lot of money and time into the house that we were trying to help her sell. Had Kate and the kids moved back into that house it most likely never would have sold and we would have lost our investment.

Charley and I had also adopted our seven year old grandson, Eddie. The years of living with epilepsy should have taught me what the chaos created by three small children living with us could do to Charley mentally. If I did not fully recognize the potential problems clusters of seizures can cause I doubt someone unfamiliar with seizures would have a clue. I do not know what we could have done differently. We would not have let our children be homeless because of Charley having seizures. We worked very hard to live as normally as possible. Taking care of our daughter during her crisis was normal for our family.

Our goal was accomplished when Kate's house sold after a few months. She had enough money to pay all her debt and purchase another home. We diligently began looking for a house. She found the perfect house and signed a contract for the purchase. Charley was having clusters of seizures (we did not know then what clusters of seizures were) with the chaos in our home multiplying the problem. Charley was mentally hanging on by a thread and stated it was all he could do to handle the situation. I thought I understood how he felt because it was all I could do to live with the situation too. A year of two families sharing one roof is difficult. We were all anxious to get back to normal.

The house Kate signed a contract on was for sale by a man who had recently divorced. The court ordered him to sell the house and give his ex-wife her share of the proceeds After a few weeks it was obvious the sale was a show and the homeowner never intended to sell the house.

Kate and I went back to square one but Charley could not. The fake sale pushed him into a major episode of psychosis. I tried to convince him everything was going to be alright but clusters of seizures were pushing him beyond the grasp of reality.

The situation was very traumatic. He was pacing around in the house and the next thing I knew he had a gun in each hand. Eventually he, Kate and I wound up in our closet because that is where all of his guns were and we were trying to keep the guns out of the situation. Kate and I should have run out of the house but instead we confronted Charley in an attempt to halt his behavior. Insane atmospheres do not create sound decisions. We were trying to slow Charley down but our attempts failed. Kate and I ended up bruised and bloody before Charley broke away from us and ran outside crazily clutching a loaded gun in each hand.

Charley ran outside and put the guns in the trunk of the car. At that time I was locking him out of the house. He came to our patio doors and became enraged when he realized he could not get back in the house. He began beating on the door with a large cinder block and destroyed the knob and deadbolt. Kate and I hid the kids before Charley broke through the door and reentered the house. I had called the sheriff. Soon after Charley broke back into the house deputies arrived and put him in the police car. I remember him sitting in the back seat looking at me with the eyes of a lost child saying, "I guess we are over now." I told Charley everything would be alright and cried like a baby when they drove away.

I had lived with Charley's epilepsy more than twenty years when this took place. Eventually a similar situation would have occurred whether Kate lived with us or not because Charley's psychosis was becoming constant. In my heart I knew seizures caused his behavior, but I did not fully understand psychosis. In other words, I knew Charley could not help what he did but I still thought he should somehow be capable of making choices. At this time I had never heard of clusters of seizures or postictal psychosis. I was confused, physically and mentally exhausted, bloody, bruised and tired of the entire situation. For the first time I came very close to giving up. Quitting cannot last long when your sick husband has been hauled off to jail.

I called David and Cheryl and told them what happened. When she asked me why all I could say is because Charley is crazy. They came to our house and helped me sort through my emotions until I could think rationally. David found the guns and unloaded them. Kate and I were angry until David's rational thinking and great respect for Charley forced us to put the situation into perspective. First David said, "Charley is sick, period." I needed to hear someone who knew about Charley's behavior say those words. David also firmly stated, "Charley would never, ever, ever hurt you or anyone else unless he was sick."

After over twenty years of hiding Charley's behavior I cried and told my family the truth. Kate called Denton, who is a close friend of ours, and he came to our house. In the past we lived next door to Denton and his wife Lynnette for thirteen years. On numerous occasions they helped me during seizure events. Though Denton saw us on a daily basis he had no clue of the occasional terror Charley's psychosis created. I did a very good of a job hiding our secrets. Those years of battling an unnamed enemy landed us at the point of no return.

We had to get Charley out of jail. It was only a matter of time before he would have tonic-clonic seizures. David called the sheriff and explained the situation and Charley was granted an emergency medical bond. David and Cheryl gathered up the only money any of us had which was the one and five dollar bills that were supposed to go into their cash register when they opened the restaurant the next day. They gave Denton the money and he went to the jail and counted out one dollar bill after one dollar bill to the jailer (whom Denton jokingly told he was a drug dealer and that's where all the one dollar bills came from) to pay Charley's five hundred dollar bail. Charley went home with Denton and stayed there for several weeks until Kate and the kids moved. Denton took great care of Charley and I am forever grateful for his kindness.

The next agenda was to find Charley medical help. After a brief search on the internet I found that the University of Texas Southwestern Medical Center in Dallas, Texas had a clinic that specialized in epilepsy. Dallas was about a six hour drive from our home and not too far to take Charley. As I weighed our options I read that their goal is to help patients become seizure free. I doubted Charley would ever be without seizures but I called and explained his situation and immediately an appointment was made with a neurologist, Dr. Diaz-Arrastia. Our point of no return quickly landed us at the beginning of a new journey.

Eventually the domestic violence charges that were filed against Charley due to this violent episode were dropped because of a letter Dr. Diaz-Arrastia wrote to the county attorney explaining that clusters of seizures and postictal psychosis had created the situation. That letter, written in 2002 confirmed my suspicions about Charley's behavior being a product of seizures and provided answers to questions that I had been asking since 1980 .

A few months later I made an appointment with the sheriff and took him a copy of the letter. I thought explaining the situation was the best way to ensure Charley was not arrested if I ever needed help due to another psychotic episode. The sheriff said if I called again for help Charley would be arrested, regardless of his medical circumstances. I numbly walked out of his office and thought to myself, "this is exactly why I never asked anyone for help." Who would believe me if I told them Charley's problems were caused by seizures? A letter written by a doctor explaining Charley's medical situation presented to the sheriff (someone who should be intelligent enough to understand the situation) meant nothing.

When you have faith you cannot let doubt creep into your soul and destroy what you know to be true. I had faith in Charley and knew he was a good person whose behavior was somehow related to his epilepsy but could find no answers. I did not tell our secrets because no one would have believed me. I kept my faith strong and we both endured a horrible illness because of a lack of decipherable information.

Some doctors assert in medical papers that psychosis is common and others proclaim it to be a rare. Lets figure psychosis out and help others who are hiding and suffering. The time is long past for everyone to be educated about clusters of seizures and every type of psychosis that those seizures can create.

Chapter 16

Our Journey to Surgery

Charley and I led an interesting life. During the first few years of our marriage except for his unpredictable behavior due to occasional bouts of psychosis our life was normal. We both worked steadily to maintain our household. Charley had seizures and job losses due to his bad memory and surly attitude but we survived and grew as a couple.

Gosh, looking back it seems time has flown by. Charley has been dead a year and I a widow. I reflect on the years we spent together and honestly cannot remember when we went from a loving couple who dealt with occasional seizures to Charley always being a sick man and I his full-time care taker. We evolved. Our life evolved. Charley's epilepsy evolved and his erratic behavior occurred more often.

We enjoyed the years we spent together raising our children. Charley's psychosis was always present and created problems as the kids grew older. Our children and I knew something was wrong with Charley. When he acted unjustly and no sense could be made of his motives we looked the other way and pushed aside our feelings and damaged emotions for the sake of keeping peace. Charley statements were often wrong but it was evident that he completely believed himself as he explained one or another incident that had taken place between him and the kids. I told our children that I knew they were being truthful but I could not assert that Charley was lying. In his mind he was telling the truth his damaged brain believed. Throughout their lives each of our children found Charley crumpled up lying somewhere, often amid his tools, from an unexpected seizure.

The years progressed and our children left home. Charley and I were together twenty-four hours a day seven days a week and we did well. We had few arguments because I knew the rules that the psychosis had created. Out of respect for Charley's needs I tried to follow those rules.

Charley and I enjoyed our time together building our beautiful two-story house, his greatest dream in life. I wanted to see his dream come true so badly that I quit college (my greatest dream in life) to help. Charley's behavior often left doubts about his skill as a carpenter to those who did not know him. Building our house was his way of mooning the world.

We inherited land from my mother and knew the only way we would ever have a nice home was to build it. We were both skilled at carpentry and construction and managed, mostly with David and Cheryl's help (other family did pitch in some) to dig trenches, set forms, run the plumbing and pour the slab. It took Charley and I two years sunup to sundown to finish building an amazing house. Not a bad accomplishment for a carpenter who happened to have seizures and his faithful helper.

Charley showed his strengths by accomplishing a monumental task most healthy people would never begin to embark upon. However; those two years of constant work took a final toll that he never recovered from. The entire time Charley was building the house he pushed seizures away with all the strength his mind could muster. A few times seizures took over but for the most part he was pretty healthy. The brain work he did to accomplish finishing his dream left little room for seizures to steal the day.

After the carpet was laid and we stopped working on a daily list of projects Charley's brain crashed. He began having seizures daily. We rocked along for about a year and then Kate and the kids moved in which turned out to be more than he could withstand.

My Charley, who had been getting up early and working late became a man who could barely drag himself out of bed and get dressed. The back of his head wore holes in the headrest of our recliner from him sitting in the same chair day after day. He was unable to accomplish anything due to being worn out beyond any capacity that a damaged brain could overcome.

We accomplished Charley's dream and life turned into a nightmare. After his psychotic episode that sent him to jail it was past time to find qualified medical help. When I told Charley we were going to consult with doctors in Dallas he adamantly stated he did not want anyone cutting his head open. What? I thought his mentioning brain surgery at that time was absurd. Who said anything about cutting his head open? I just wanted to get his seizures under control. We agreed other avenues had to be explored so I drove Charley to Dallas to consult with Dr Diaz-Arrastia.

After we arrived at the clinic in Dallas I filled out the new patient information sheet. I wrote "Daily seizures - falling down and urinating on self. Tooth grinding at night – wandering combative emotional seizures to the point of being a danger to others and self. Grand Mal seizures occur at least 4 – 5 times a month. Severe depression and the possibility of dementia – has symptoms. Constant seizures must be damaging the brain. Help – We need help!" I now know those emotional seizures were actually clusters of seizures and being combative was caused by psychosis.

Charley's mind was weak and body tired but we were on the right track taking him to epilepsy specialists. I was surprised when Charley immediately announced to Dr. Diaz-Arrastia that he was ready to have anything done, including having his head cut open, to get the seizures under control and regain his life. What? When Charley made that statement I almost told him to quit joking. My husband was more intelligent than I ever will be.

I was skeptical when Dr. Diaz-Arrastia stated his goal was to see Charley become seizure free. I could not imagine our life without seizures ruling every moment. The doctor prescribed a medication that controlled the seizures for a couple of months. In time the seizures broke through the medication and we were back to square one. We returned to Dallas and another medication was prescribed. Within a couple of weeks Charley began having multiple seizures. Between the old and new medications and constant seizures Charley's brain was only operating at about fifty percent. I described him as living in loony land because he was always highly agitated and could not distinguish reality from imagination. Charley could not remember he had a doctor's appointment or drive himself anywhere. I was fully responsible for the life of a man I dearly loved. No words can accurately describe my fear.

After seizures broke through the second medication Dr. Diaz-Arrastia suggested that Charley begin a series of tests to see if he might be a candidate for brain surgery. The doctor told us if the tests went well we might have a hope of eliminating seizures altogether. Charley swallowed a huge lump in his throat and agreed to the tests. We later returned to Dallas for an on-camera observation of his seizures in the Epilepsy Unit at Parkland Hospital. An E.E.G. was hooked up to Charley. Small round disks were glued to his head by a pretty technician. He flirted with her as she explained how the E.E.G. would pinpoint the area in his brain where the seizures occurred. Previous tests had located his seizures in the left temporal lobe and the E.E.G. confirmed this. If the seizures originated in his left temporal lobe and crossed over to the right side of his brain he would have been eliminated as a surgery candidate. We were told that a person whose seizures cross over from one side of the brain to the other loses their chance at surgery during this first step. Only one temporal lobe can be removed.

We stayed in a small room in the epilepsy unit. Charley had a hospital bed and I a small couch to sleep on. After the E.E.G. was hooked up his medications were withheld and a camera was constantly aimed at him in order to observe potential seizures. If he moved anywhere the camera followed. The nurses told us many people who have seizures check into the epilepsy unit for observation and do not have a seizure. Charley just looked at the nurses and I told them to give us a couple of hours and the show would begin. Shortly afterward Charley had his first on-camera seizure. I had to push a button to alert the nurses of the seizure. My focus was always on keeping Charley safe when he had a seizure so the button messed up my rhythm.

The room quickly filled with medical staff. For the first time in over twenty years I had qualified people helping me through one of Charley's seizures. I did not have to protect him. They understood seizures and complimented me for the way I took care of my husband. I was surrounded by people who said they admired me for the love I showed Charley and the care I gave. I felt someone understood my burdens. I drew much strength from their support. Charley had several seizures over a thirty-six hour observation period and was placed back on his medication.

Prior to being released Charley underwent a psychiatric evaluation. I was scuttled out of the room by the doctor who told me the exam would take a couple of hours. The doctor suggested I go shopping.

I was driving our twelve year old clunker van that David had to put Freon in before every trip so the air conditioner would work. That van took us to Dallas and got us home because that's what God wanted. I was not real sure God wanted me to go shopping so for several hours my fear and I sat alone in the van in the dark parking garage of the hospital while Charley underwent his psychiatric tests. I did not expect Charley to pass the evaluation but he did. Upon reading medical records after Charley died I discovered the psychiatrists who did this evaluation diagnosed Charley as having hallucinations and hearing voices. I should have been informed of this fact but was not. The psychiatric doctors may have thought I knew.

Each step toward brain surgery led to a team of doctors holding a conference to discuss Charley's case and decide if we could move forward. After our experiences I strongly suggest to anyone pursuing brain surgery and undergoing these types of tests to make sure you read and are aware of the results of every test. Acquire the facts and get the paperwork and use that information to make your decision of whether or not to proceed with the next step and eventual brain surgery.

Charley's last test in order to qualify as a good surgery candidate was called a Wada. I scheduled the test but initially cancelled because we were broke and I was scared. The trips to Dallas and expense of the new medicine were beyond our means. I kept holding on to a false hope that Charley would miraculously improve. We knew how to deal with seizures but had no idea what might be impaired due to the surgery. I felt whatever abilities Charley lost would be my fault because I had taken him to the doctors in Dallas.

Day in and day out I obsessed about the potential results of Charley undergoing brain surgery. The previous twenty-two years of my life were spent protecting Charley. I drove him everywhere he needed to go. I caught him when he fell and cleaned him when he had seizures. I hid his psychosis, babied him when he was sick, often held him while he cried. Protecting Charley was my life. I mentally slammed into stone walls as I tried to determine what was more important to protect Charley from; seizures or brain surgery?

What would be best? I knew Charley would suffer some degree of loss with either decision. Would it be best for him to continue to have seizures or for him to have his temporal lobe removed? Would he lose some of his speech, mental abilities, memory and normal functions? What if he suffered these losses and still had seizures? I was not sure he had the mental strength to withstand the results of surgery if it did not stop the seizures. Charley was not capable of making a decision about surgery alone. I did not want to push him in any direction that might cause more harm than good.

Oh . . . My God . . . I was scared.

A few months rocked along and Charley did fairly well on his new medications for a man who had seizures all the time. We were comfortable with our misery but I knew every seizure was eating away at his brain. We hoped for improvement but seizures were stealing our life. I made another appointment with Dr. Diaz-Arrastia and drove Charley to Dallas.

During this visit Dr. Diaz-Arrastia said Charley was a great candidate for surgery and explained to him that he was having clusters of seizures seven days a week twenty-four hours a day. Dr. Diaz-Arrastia felt their medical team could help and he sincerely wanted to give Charley a seizure-free life. He asked Charley to go through with the Wada test so we could complete the process and establish him as a surgery candidate. Charley agreed to the test and it was time for me to swallow the huge lump in my throat. I had to put aside my fear in order to positively support Charley through this journey. We were passing another point of no return. How damn many of those is one couple supposed to endure in a lifetime?

We came home and the test was scheduled for a few weeks later and again, David forced Freon in the air conditioner of our clunker van and we returned to Dallas. The Wada test, officially known as the intracarotid sodium amobarbital test looks at memory and language functions by putting one cerebral hemisphere to sleep with a short-acting anesthetic and studying what functions are still working in the other hemisphere. The test begins with an angiogram which examines the flow of a dye through the blood vessels. A catheter is introduced through an artery in the inner portion of the upper thigh. A local anesthetic is given to numb the area and a needle is then inserted into the artery. The tube is threaded through the needle, and the needle is removed. There is some mild discomfort during the local anesthesia but the rest of the test is painless. The tube is guided up to the carotid artery in the neck. A small amount of contrast dye is injected through the tube into the artery and x-rays are taken to study the flow of blood in the brain. Next, the radiologist injects amobarbital which puts almost half of the cerebral hemisphere to sleep for several minutes. Immediately after the injection tests are given to see how well language and memory are working with half of the brain sleeping. This provides information on the functions of the cerebral hemisphere that is sleeping and the hemisphere that is awake. The same procedure is usually repeated on the opposite side after a delay (one half to one hour or sometimes a day) to ensure that the patient's level of alertness has returned to normal. Charley had some pain and discomfort from the test but passed with no problem.

After Charley was dismissed from the hospital I drove home with my mental capacities in slow motion. I steadily kept the van at the speed limit as my fears slowly processed. Charley was almost insane. He kicked the walls of the van as he lay on the bed in the back and tearfully told me he would not blame me if I left him while I was ahead. What? (In my mind I wondered what in the hell is ahead? If this situation puts me ahead someone please shoot me now). Charley said he would rather be dead than mentally out of control and have to watch himself be crazy with no way of reigning himself in. I could only listen. I felt so bad for Charley and any words spoken added to his grief.

When we got home and Charley settled into his worn recliner I gave him time to calm down and then sat on his lap facing him with my knees tucked between his legs and the arms of the chair. I rubbed Charley's goatee, looked straight into his beautiful blue eyes and slowly moved my face closer and closer to him until my nose softly touched his. I put my hands on his cheeks, gave him a soft kiss and spoke gently but forcefully as I wanted to get beyond his mental anguish and sooth his insecurities. I told Charley it was not easy living with his seizures but in no way did I blame him. We held each others hands tightly. Tears streamed down both of our faces as we looked into each others eyes and came to grips with our fears. I promised Charley I would never leave. We would remain together in sickness and in health until death as we promised in our wedding vows.

I reminded Charley of the love and devotion he had shown while taking care of me after three surgeries I had endured during our years together. We laughed through our tears as I reminisced about a time I was trying to get dressed after having had back surgery. I stood in our bedroom wearing only a back brace with my panties hanging loosely around my ankles. I called to Charley and asked him to come pull my panties up as I was in too much pain to bend over. He came in our bedroom and distressfully said, "I can't, I can't. I only know how to pull your panties down."

We agreed the unknowns of brain surgery were very frightening but knew Charley would not be functioning much longer if he kept having seizures. Together we were backed into a corner and the only hope we had of getting out was brain surgery. I told Charley, "We never let epilepsy defeat us. Brain surgery is not going to defeat us either." I cannot imagine any couple facing brain surgery without fear.

We united our attitudes and from that moment on created determination from our fear and moved forward without wasting time looking back. Charley seldom voiced his fears, though I know he felt them often. Once in a while fear would creep into my soul and nearly bring me to my knees. I told myself if he can do this, then I can do this. I wiped the involuntary tears terror instantly creates out of my eyes and forced myself to draw strength from my husband's determination.

Charley told our friends and family the doctors in Dallas had found the reason for his seizures. His story was he had way too much brain and that is what caused him to be smarter than everyone else. The mystery was solved! He said the doctors were going to remove some of his brain to eliminate seizures but not to worry. He reassured everyone that he would remain smarter than them and in no way would removing a small extra piece of his brain alter the fact that he was perfect! With the never-ending support of our family and friends Mr. Perfect and I began the next steps of our journey.

I had to find a way to pay for these trips and mounting medical bills. When we were at home every spare minute was spent selling everything collectible that we owned on E-bay. Whatever fit into a box and could be shipped went up for auction. We sold antique marbles, bottles, beads, toy cars, books, fishing poles, skis, life jackets, jewelry, tools and numerous other items. Listing items on E-bay was something we could do together in the confines of our home. When Charley fell over having seizures, which occurred pretty darned often, I rolled him off of the items we were going to sell that were piled all over the floor and diligently continued selling our old life to fund a new one.

Our next assignment was to find a mental health physician for Charley to consult with after surgery. We made an appointment at the Veterans Hospital in Amarillo and their doctors agreed to see him, completed paperwork and sent it to the medical team in Dallas.

Next we traveled back to Dallas to meet Charley's assigned brain surgeon, Dr. Bruce Mickey. He asked Charley if he realized how many medical staff it had taken and how much work they had done to get him to the point that he was meeting with a brain surgeon. Dr. Mickey told Charley the medical team had done their job and it was time that he did his which was to quit smoking cigarettes. Dr. Mickey is a very intelligent man who knew how to respectfully address Charley, skirt around his complicated medical problems, and quickly earn his return respect. It took a lot to make a demand of Charley and get results but he did quit smoking because surgery was much more important to him than cigarettes.

We met once again with Dr. Mickey and Charley's surgery was scheduled for June 7th of 2004. Our long time friend, John Bevers (J.B.) had unexpectedly died the previous year and June 7th was his birthday – the day meant for Charley's surgery. We had no one to accompany us to Dallas for Charley's surgery but I was never alone. Knowing JB's spirit was there was very comforting.

We pulled our homely green and white camper behind our beat-up brown and gold van (that David had kindly put Freon in again) and left for Dallas a week early. I wanted to spend quality time together before surgery. Angela, our niece who lived near Dallas, took us to the rodeo. Charley loved the rodeo and told me I could keep spoiling him as long as I wanted.

We went to the hospital to pre-register and meet with the staff who would attend the surgery. Every staff member asked Charley if he knew what surgery they were going to perform. His answer was correct; brain surgery. My scared mind kept asking my heavy heart how we had gotten to this place in our life. Did we do something wrong? Could we have prevented Charley needing surgery by some unknown action that we had never discovered? I was so sad. The night before surgery sleep eluded us both as we cried and made love all night. We softly touched each other and whispered our fears as we said our good-byes to the life we had known for over twenty years.

Early the next morning we arrived at the hospital and checked in. Charley was exhausted and overwhelmed by fear. The staff was gathered and Charley prepped for surgery. I felt my soul laying on the gurney with my husband as he was rolled away. I handed God my doubt and fear and sat alone in the waiting room with a spiral notebook and captured my feelings for this book. This is what I wrote:

June 7th, 2004

"If anyone asked me to describe epilepsy in one word the word would be alone. Like a tree that is standing far off in the distance overshadowed by a cloudy sky. That is epilepsy. Misunderstood, misinterpreted, stumbling through life in a world not even understood by the very person living it; alone. I sit in a surgery waiting room after 24 years of epilepsy ruling mine and my husband's life. Even hope petrifies us and leaves us alone.

Epilepsy is such an unknown illness. Just a word, always hope someone will understand. The few people that do become a part of the person who has epilepsy's life are very special. Most people aren't willing to take the time to step into someone else's life. A person with epilepsy is like a lone survivor on an island far, far in the middle of the ocean . . . alone . . . alone.

Throughout our life many people have paddled out to our island, visited, come and gone. Eventually, usually, they stay out of the canoe, lose the paddles, and just go away. Who wants to swim in a sea of misunderstanding? It takes special people with special love to endure friendship with someone who has epilepsy.

What do you do and how do you help? Do you have a family member who has epilepsy and you feel you cannot go away? Well, believe me, you can. Many members of Charley's family have trickled away over the years. Mostly because they don't understand this illness and rather than listen they run and blame. Where to begin? I only know one story: the story of Charley and Lola. But the epilepsy stretches back to his childhood, I am sure. I cannot prove the origins of his illness but I think from the many talks we have had that he started life with epilepsy.

Childhood:

Charley was raised in a children's home from the age of five. He remembers being in a vehicle with his older brother and sister and singing as they were being taken away from their parents and transported to the children's home. Charley's parents were separated and unable to take care of the children so at a young age Charley was introduced to a very structured environment. This was good as a character builder but bad as a comparison factor.

A little boy that cannot think correctly in a home with thirty two little boys that can. A little boy that can't remember, forgets instructions, and was probably walking into walls half of the time. Charley was in trouble a lot and this little boy who needed special attention was cheated severely by his life circumstances.

However, I doubt at that time anyone could have recognized Charley's epilepsy. I imagine someone knew something was not right but I doubt they realized something was wrong. I bet he had episodes of staring or dozing as a child and was frequently lost, even in familiar environments. We were told by Charley's mother that he had seizures when he had high fever as a child. This was a huge thing to learn. To me this is a link from this surgery waiting room all the way back to Charley's childhood.

It is a hell of a feeling to wait for someone to have surgery to help this illness. What if this surgery does not help? Can this poor man endure this surgery if it fails? I wanted to tell the doctor fix Charley or kill him. Of course that is an irrational thought. I don't want my husband to die. I just want him to live, really live like a normal human being. I want him to not be alone.

When Charley had his first Grand Mal Seizure in front of me I had no idea what to do. This was our second date, we were going to go dancing – wham – Charley hit the floor and had a huge seizure. I had always heard the tongue could be swallowed so I stuck my finger in his mouth to hold his tongue down.

Well, the focus quickly changed from Charley having a seizure to I have to save my finger and quite frankly I was a lot more worried about my finger than I was Charley. Finally, after a good minute, his bite unlocked and I retrieved my purple, tooth-marked finger. I did not learn what to do about a seizure but I learned one thing not to do. An ambulance was summoned and the doctor in the emergency room prescribed dilantin and sent us on our way. We each had thousands of questions and no one to answer them.

Over and over during this journey Charley and I have asked why. I suggest a time limit to wonder why and then go on. I am sure a lot of people who have epilepsy know the root cause of the seizures, perhaps accidents or illness. However, knowing the root cause does not answer why, it only answers how and I cannot see any comfort from that. A person facing epilepsy has the right to ask why but don't expect an answer. Asking why has put us on the receiving end of strange looks from more doctors than can be imagined.

Don't strand yourself on a deserted island with alone and why. This leads to horrid depression. Why does not matter and is a stumbling block that can get a person down more than seizures. Put why aside. Life will answer the question of why as you face every obstacle epilepsy puts in front of you.

Now I am waiting to see Charley. His left temporal lobe has been removed. What a stone to the heart to have a doctor tell you, "We took out the left temporal lobe, that entire part of Charley's brain." The words we are and the words we have certainly create different lumps in the throat. Will Charley know me? Will he still love me? Will he be angry? Will he be weak on one side? So many questions but I am not asking why. It is up from here. Up, Up, Up!

That is what I wrote as I waited for Charley to come out of surgery.

Dr. Mickey came in the waiting room and talked to me about the surgery and assured me everything had gone well. I told him Charley would be fine because he is a very strong man. Dr. Mickey told me, "Yes, and Charley has a very strong wife." I never forgot that compliment.

Shortly afterward I was allowed to see Charley in the intensive care unit, but was told in no uncertain terms I could not stay (here we go again). I respected the hospital's rules but told the nurse if Charley needed to be calmed I was the person for the job. I stood at the end of the bed intently watching his every move. He lifted his right arm and it was weak and shaky. As Charley lifted his arm I could practically see his brain trying to figure out what had just happened. If his brain could have spoken the thoughts it was processing at that moment it would have asked, "Where is the part of me that runs this arm?"

I was observing Charley as his brain tried to make his right arm work correctly. I saw a slow but smooth transition take place as his arm began to work. He lifted his right arm again and about half-way up the shaking stopped, weakness disappeared, and the arm worked fine. Next I watched Charley's right leg and it began to lift off of the bed. I was observing an "all systems check" that was happening. His right leg was weak and shaky when he first tried to lift it but within seconds I believe his brain re-routed its signals and his leg quit shaking and worked fine. Charley looked at me and said, "Hi sugar." I cried with relief and kissed him and told him how proud I was that he was so strong. Shortly afterward I was asked to leave because my visiting time was over. Once again I told the nurses if Charley needed to be calmed I was the person for the job.

Sometime within the next hour a nurse asked me to return to Charley's room. I do not know what happened. Charley was always very dramatic when in pain. His arms and legs were tied to the bed and he was yelling and cursing his discomfort. Oh, I was so glad to hear those familiar words and honestly wanted him to keep shouting. Every expletive Charley loudly grumbled revealed how much of my surly husband was coming home with me. The nurses wanted nothing more than to find a way to get him quiet while I was reveling in every word he loudly uttered. I talked to Charley and reassured him and in a matter of minutes I untied his legs and arms. He calmly slept as I sat by his side and rubbed his hand. No more throwing me out of the room (as usual). I was a welcome intruder.

I did not stay the entire night but waited to leave until I knew he would be alright. I told Charley I was leaving and made him promise to behave. I desperately needed time to myself in order to gather my strength and face the next day. I returned to our camper and listened to Hank Williams Sr. music that soothed my soul. To this day I cannot hear any of those songs without crying.

The next morning when I walked into the hospital room I asked Charley how he felt. He grimaced and said, "Quit yelling, Lo, I am not deaf."

Initially I did not comprehend what he was telling me and I teasingly said, "Oh, yes you are." (Before surgery he was partially deaf in both ears and wore hearing aids).

Charley said, "No, I am not deaf. I can hear just fine. I hear everyone's voice that has spoken to me. I am not deaf anymore."

I was stunned. One part of me thought he was kidding and the other part knew he was serious. "Charley, are you serious? You can hear?" I asked him.

"Yes, I can hear fine and you are going to have to quit talking so damn loud." he replied. His voice was lower and quieter and hearing completely restored.

Charley avoided talking on the telephone for several years prior because his loss of hearing was frustrating. Lying in that hospital bed with two black eyes and his face swollen up like a car had run over his head one of Charley's greatest joys was speaking to our friends and family on the telephone and actually hearing their voices. Our family was stunned when I told them Charley could hear.

"He can hear?" they asked me.

"Yes, he can hear. Talk to him. You won't believe this." I told everyone.

No one really wanted to talk to Charley on the telephone because they did not want him frustrated. In the past they had to shout and he usually still could not understand. I handed him the phone and made everyone talk to him so they would believe me. We were amazed by Charley instantly regaining the ability to hear. Not everyone walking on this planet can say they have truly witnessed a miracle.

When I told Cheryl that Charley could hear she was the only person who did not hesitate to want to speak to him. She immediately said, "Oh, bull, that old fart cannot hear a damn thing. Hand him the phone." Charley put the phone up to his ear and quickly pulled it away as Cheryl almost deafened him for life when she yelled, "Can you hear me you old fart? Faked not being able to hear for years just to get attention didn't you?"

Charley replied, "Hell yes, you old bag. And it worked too! I had you fooled!"

Some things never change.

Charley did very well after surgery and immediately wanted to come home. I knew he was going to have horrendous headaches and wanted him to stay on an IV painkiller. He did not have a bad headache until three days after surgery. Charley pleaded with every doctor that came in the room to let him go home. He got his way and was scheduled for dismissal on the fourth day after surgery. Charley checked out of the hospital and we went to our camper to spend the night. It had been raining in Dallas and our camper was infested with black ants that were looking for a dry home.

Charley became very sick with a horrible headache and threw up all night. I took care of him and kept the ants off of him the best I could. The next morning while he slept I hooked the van to the camper and then helped him get from the camper to the bed in the van. We headed home. I do not know if anyone can imagine what it would be like to have your face cut open and peeled away from your temple on Monday, holes drilled in your skull, part of your brain removed and the following Saturday ride in a bouncing, worn out van that is pulling a camper for six hours before arriving home. The trip was torture. I was exhausted and cried most of the way because I could do nothing to help with Charley's misery. I honestly think the trip caused him at least an extra week of agony.

We arrived home and Charley went to bed. Our beautiful, quiet house wrapped its welcoming arms around us as we began a new journey through Charley's healing.

Chapter 17

Healing, Progression and Insanity after Surgery

Of all the chapters I have revised this one has been the most difficult. My sole intent of writing is to help others whose journeys take them down the same roads we traveled. I could leave out a few of the following pages and no one would know our hardships after Charley's surgery. Or, I can speak the truth but along with that comes the burden of potentially frightening others.

Thousands of vehicles drive down highways without having accidents. Occasionally, on the very roads we travel, a crash occurs that results in severe injuries or fatalities. Knowing an accident happened does not mean we forever avoid driving down that road. The scene of an accident reminds us to be careful as we travel, but the course we set and roads we travel do not change.

Charley's epilepsy before surgery was extreme and after surgery his case followed protocol. Though most never will, a small percentage of people who have seizures eliminated through surgery could have the same problems. Sugar-coating these events is intentionally choosing to withhold information from people who may need it. It is easy to be swallowed by situations and have no clue what to do when living within darkness that is created by the unknown. Do not let that happen to you in any circumstance epilepsy creates.

This book is not written with the intent of swaying anyone from the road they are traveling if that road leads to brain surgery eliminating seizures. The only way to present our circumstances is truthfully. I can rework the words but there is no justification for setting aside the original reasons for this book. Brain surgery did not immediately make our life easy. The end result of having Charley's seizures eliminated through surgery is the good positively outweighed the bad a million to one, it just took a while to get there.

If you are fortunate enough to be on the way to having seizures eliminated through surgery stay on that road. I would give anything if the following events never happened, but they did. I write the truth to help others be aware and careful during their journeys, not to sway anyone's course.

Our Journey After Surgery

Charley was miserable with severe headaches for a couple of months. I took care of him like a child. While he numbly sat naked in the bathtub and let me wash his body I told him I bathed him so he would know he was still alive.

"Dead people don't take baths, Charley." I whispered.

For several weeks he laid on the living room floor all day, more miserable with his body on a bed or couch than he was on the floor. Seeing him lying on the floor as he endured horrible pain broke my heart. Charley was tying his entire being to the earth and letting the natural flow of the world enter his system in order to stay calm, endure the pain and allow his brain to heal.

Charley was a very strong man who had been mentally fighting seizures for years and now they were gone. The minute he woke from surgery we both knew he would never have another seizure. We were again exploring uncharted territory. Hour upon hour I sat in our living room with Charley, watching him not have seizures, as he slept on the floor and endured the headaches. He was undoubtedly in pain, but a new man whose face was relaxed and eyes clear. For the first time in years Charley was not struggling with a locomotive running through his head, not mentally fighting seizures and no longer driven by a constant push in a mind that never rested. As I kept watch I tried in thousands of ways to convince myself that our hard times were over. My heart refused to listen. Many years of living with seizures had taught me that no gains are made without paying a price. I stared at my new husband as tears rolled down my cheeks and continually prayed to find the peace and happiness we both deserved.

I passed time wondering what had that little piece of brain the doctors removed contained. Would Charley still be my carpenter man? Would he know what a hammer was and be able to drive a nail? I wanted to hold tools in front of him and ask if he knew what they were. But I did not. I impatiently waited for him to take steps in this new life in his own time.

As Charley's headaches decreased he moved from the floor to the couch and after several weeks began sitting in his chair. It seemed he had been wearing pajamas forever. About six weeks after surgery he walked downstairs wearing jeans, a tee shirt and carrying a pair of socks. Tears ran down my face. Everything scared me to death.

I asked Charley, "What are you doing?"

He said, "I don't know; something."

It does not take much to be something when you have been living with seizures as a couple for over twenty years and then gone through brain surgery. Seeing him dressed was a huge something. He put on his socks and shoes and went out the front door.

I sat like a stone looking through our glass storm door and watched Charley walk toward his shop. I had to allow him to start fresh and enjoy a new beginning. I wanted to follow and ask a million questions to see what he remembered. I left him and his new brain alone. A few hours later a very tired Charley came into the house and took a nap. While he slept I went to the shop to see what he had done. Tools were organized that had been lying dusty and unused for more than a year before surgery.

Life rocked along and Charley puttered around keeping busy on small projects. He was physically weak because constant seizures had prevented activity. Overworking caused severe headaches. We stuck to our list system and I tried to pace him, however; that was very difficult because of a two-fold problem. Charley's thoughts were severely obsessive (worrying uncontrollably about a particular thing, or things) and he was extremely compulsive (his actions were driven by an unusually irrational psychological force).

Charley healed for a couple of months and it became apparent he had a distance (in his mind) from reality that he did not understand (in his heart) as mental instability. In many ways his surgery was mentally as hard on me as him. I had a distance from reality (in my mind) that I did understand (in my heart) that had been created by years of conditioning I endured in order to live with Charley's sporadic psychotic behavior. The left temporal lobe of his brain was removed which apparently was not only the seizure location but also contained whatever caused his psychosis. For more than twenty years I had lived with ugly moods and met unreasonable expectations during psychotic episodes. I was conditioned to walk on eggshells in order to maintain some semblance of sanity while we endured his insanity.

Charley came out of surgery a completely different person. The surgeons cut out a piece of his brain and along with that piece of brain went his clusters of seizures and postictal psychosis. His mind could not remember events that my heart would not forget. I had danced around psychosis and hardened my spirit to the point that no ugly words could wound me. My inner being instantly knew phrases that were the first sign of an episode of psychosis. I was mentally conditioned to shut down normal instant defensive reactions most people have when verbally assaulted. When Charley was psychotic due to seizures I did not defend myself. The first action I trained myself to take when it became apparent that my Charley was no longer present and his psychosis had taken over was to confront him with my eyes. When Charley started into a round of psychosis my hackles instantly rose upon hearing distinct phrases. I was mentally trained to emotionally shut down and whispered to myself, "That is not Charley." When he was suffering from psychosis he never heard me whisper out loud. He was in motion, pacing, cursing, threatening, and slamming doors. I was the opposite; calm, still, quiet, and observant.

I had a huge problem after Charley's surgery. He did not know the words that had once signaled the beginning of a psychotic episode, but my inner being did. He began to feel good and could converse with me (especially in the mornings). He innocently said something familiar from our past insanity that never meant anything to him and my panic emerged, hackles rose, emotions shut down and the gates within my heart that only allowed a nice Charley inside instantly closed. I immediately put on my mental armor and shut down emotionally to not needlessly battle with Charley's psychosis. After surgery he no longer experienced psychosis and was totally puzzled by my reactions. He asked, "What in the hell is the matter with you?" and blankly stared at me in the same way I must have stared at him for years.

Charley did not remember past psychosis and I could not explain the mental suffering or conditioning I endured. He clued-in very quickly that my present behavior was not normal. Doctors did not take me to surgery and cut out my past conditioning or survival techniques. When Charley said something that was an indicator (from the past) that psychosis was occurring I immediately started trying to calm him. Charley was calm, but I was not. I panicked and experienced the same sense of dread I felt in the past when I knew he was becoming psychotic. Within my heart was a five-hundred foot wall ready to go up so I would not be hurt by his behavior. After surgery Charley did not have the same behaviors.

But I did.

Certain distinct actions of Charley's created distinct reactions from me. Not ugly reactions but simply stated firm words I learned to use to keep him calm when he was going into a psychotic mode. His actions had been repeated and predictable and I had learned repeated predictable reactions in order to maintain a semblance of sanity in our home. I was walking on the same eggshells, adjusted to the same conditioning and living within the same protective walls time had built up within my soul. I discovered there was not much of me left. Why in the hell could not one thing in our life ever be easy?

I was stupefied.

I recognized a severe problem within myself but could not take time away from Charley to seek counseling. I observed my bizarre reactions and fearfully thought to myself, "Oh, My God!! Charley is going to be well now . . . and I am going to be crazy."

Charley held me while I cried and expressed my sorrow and apologies for my behavior. I told him how lucky he was because the surgeons cut out his previous problems and he could start a new life. My mental being was stuck in the past. Charley was different and I was the same and I could not find a way to fix myself. He wiped away my tears but did not fully comprehend my sorrow and frustration.

For the first time ever, for a short time after surgery, Charley was trying to walk on the same plane as me and damned if I could find a way to walk beside him. My emotions and mental being were beat to death. I became very depressed. Some days I felt my mind was existing among the clouds. I wondered after all the years of being a caretaker if I was somehow addicted to having a sick husband. My internal spirit did not understand how to allow us freedom from Charley's past illness.

I lost my place in life, my routine and my identity. The actions I had learned to preserve and build the best life possible for us were no longer important and were causing unbelievable stress. The elements of my personality I had trained that held me together for over twenty years were now causing me to fall apart. Literally overnight . . . the honed strengths and defense mechanisms I was so proud of . . . became weaknesses that I could not control and felt ashamed of. How hard does life have to be before you pass the test? Had I failed? I asked God to teach my lesson quickly. I needed strength and could not find any while depressed, contemplating whether or not I had in the past, or was now, failing Charley and I.

I prayed and pleaded with the Lord to help me learn to trust again. Please God, take down my walls and help us start a new life. As the days went by and I quietly whispered my prayers Charley began a new cycle of withdrawal and became mentally unstable in unfamiliar ways. I did not have time to deal with my previous conditioning before Charley's after-surgery insanity began to run rampant.

I tried to stop my conditioned responses and did well but not quickly enough. The behaviors I displayed convinced Charley that I had been the crazy one during our marriage and he had been fine. Then, dozens of times a day, he sneered at me and stated that he could "see reality." The reality he saw turned him into an obsessively mean individual determined to pay me back for a past that he could not even remember. Seizures creating his previous misery was unfathomable to Charley. There was no convincing him having a part of his brain removed might cause some irrational and unfair thoughts toward me to creep into his mind.

Charley obsessed horribly about his new found "reality" that I had always been crazy. I did not initially understand the depth of his obsession and hoped he might see some of my past sacrifices. I asked Charley if his new "reality" helped him understand how much I loved him. I wanted him to value my efforts in making sure he was the best taken care of man in the world. I told him there were lots of people wishing to be him just so they could be so loved. I asked him to please give his brain some time to heal before he condemned me as the source of all our problems. My words fell upon deaf ears. Charley's obsession was that he had always been normal and I had not. The thought that I was the cause of all our previous misery became a deeply-rooted destructive obsession within Charley's mind. He did not understand how hard I was working to change my mental being or the previous hardships caused by his psychosis. Anything I said to help him balance reality resulted in Charley sneering at me because in his mind the surgery had allowed him the ability to see how crazy I was and had always been. There was no mercy concerning the mental work I had to do to accomplish my adjustments.

"Now I see reality." Charley bitterly told me dozens of times every day. No matter how I explained the reasoning for my conditioned reactions he would never understand. The bottom line was Charley needed to heal from a very serious brain surgery. The last thing I wanted to do was torture him with facts from our past that he did not remember. He could not process my words and it was unfair to try and force him.

I want to express the physical aspect of Charley's after-surgery psychotic behavior visually in order to help with recognition. Picture an extremely obsessive person . . . thinking, thinking, thinking . . . pacing . . . on the move . . . pacing as they verbally express (to no one) over and over their thoughts or what they are on the move to do. They walk with short, fast paced steps . . . obsessively speaking their thoughts (in a monotone voice). . . almost marching without bending their knees . . . slightly leaning forward as they walk . . . struggling against an invisible wind . . . sweating without exertion. Visualize an obsessed . . . almost marching as they walk with short, fast paced steps . . . sweating person . . . whose mind is obsessively focused on fixing, finding, retrieving, hunting, cleaning, repairing, moving or destroying something or someone.

Picture that compulsive obsessed person standing behind a jet airplane and imagine turning the engine on. Do you see how intensely that person would have to work to stand up and walk and accomplish any task within such turbulence? Try to understand how hard they would have to think in order to grasp any thoughts. Can you comprehend why, once any thought was planted in their brain, that thought obsessively rooted itself deep within their mind, became an obsession, and never changed? (I see reality . . . I see reality . . . I see reality . . . I see reality).

Visualize how hard a moving, obsessed person would have to lean into the turbulence of a jet engine in order to walk. Picture a compulsive, obsessed person not only walking within such a force but their mind running full force, surrounded by the turbulence of a jet engine and not missing a beat on the way to obsessively fix, find, retrieve, hunt, clean, repair, move, destroy or tell someone whatever it is they are obsessing about. Charley was completely, totally, one hundred percent oblivious to the fact that he was surrounded by any turbulence when this obsessive behavior entirely took over his being.

This is the best I can do to provide a visual picture of the behavior Charley displayed after surgery. Initially his deeply rooted obsessive thought was "I see reality." As time passed he obsessed about other things. I believe the force that creates the behavior captures a person and takes them into a world where they honestly have no control or recollection of their actions.

I thought the behavior Charley displayed after surgery was caused by the trauma of the surgery. Dr. Mickey read the first draft of this book and disagreed. He explained the behavior with the following: "The human body is obviously far more complex than an automobile but it might help to compare Charley's combination of temporal lobe epilepsy and mental illness to a car with two separate problems: a short circuit in its electrical system and a severe problem in its cooling system. Repairing the short circuit would be expected to make the car run more smoothly, but because it was being driven greater distances than in the past, this repair might make the car overheat more frequently. The changes in Charley's behavior that you noted after his surgery probably have a similar explanation."

I have experience with one person who had brain surgery and Dr. Mickey has known hundreds and he made it very clear that Charley's case was rare. I cannot claim to know what caused his behavior to become so severe. I write about our experiences as they happened.

Before our circumstances escalated to the point I describe in this chapter I should have called the mental health doctor in Amarillo who agreed to take care of Charley. I was so confused and overcome with exhaustion that I had no common sense. Before the surgery I mistakenly thought the mental health doctor was necessary because Charley might need counseling for having lost a physical part of himself. I did not know the mental health doctor was required because there was a rare potential for Charley's behavior to become extreme. This lack of knowledge was my fault because I should have asked more questions of the doctors in Dallas prior to surgery. If you are contemplating brain surgery make an appointment to see a mental health doctor a month to six weeks after the scheduled date of surgery. I cannot stress how important it is to be prepared for both the mental and physical aspects of life after surgery.

Two to three months after surgery Charley's obsessive behavior led to threats and intimidation. He never carried out with the threats but they scared the hell out of me. Initially the episodes happened in spurts, for a few hours during the day. Eventually we suffered with irrational, obsessive behavior twenty-four hours a day seven days a week. Charley was pacing, sweating, obsessively trying to fix stuff but tearing it up, leaning against an invisible wind as he marched to nowhere like a lost soldier. He sneered at me constantly as if I were an enemy he wished to kill.

Everything Charley obsessively told me all day he obsessively repeated all night. When I became totally exhausted and tried to sleep he leapt on my bed, landed on his knees with his legs straddling me at the waist and pinned my shoulders or neck under the covers in order to make sure I was awake as he informed me that he could now see reality . . . he was normal and I was not. He continually flipped the bedroom lights on and off and paced around the house slamming doors. I struggled with trying to be patient and kind in spite of the raw fear his condition was planting within my soul. I knew Charley did not know what he was doing but exhaustion was taking its toll as neither of us had slept for many nights.

I kept thinking the behavior would level out and endured the insanity much longer than I should have. Expecting a person who has a part of their brain removed to be without problems is irrational. I knew there would be struggles but I never anticipated the situation we endured. The sleep deprivation began to prey upon my being until I was beyond comprehending what was happening. Charley marched and paced all day spurting out threats and verbally picking at me until I collapsed crying from the mental stress. He darted out the door until I had enough time to partially recover, then instantly reappeared and restarted his verbal war. Rather than go to bed at night I forced myself to stay awake and took refuge in our living room hoping to keep a safe distance between us. Charley went to the loft upstairs that overlooks our living room and threw objects down at me. I sat exhausted, praying for peace and rest, as I dodged flying shoes and pillows that were hurled at me by a madman. I tried everything to calm the insanity and nothing helped. Charley was constantly on the move - pacing inside then outside during the day - darting upstairs and downstairs during the night. He was a crazy stranger determined to intimidate me by promising to do me in because he could see reality. The beautiful home we built to enjoy our life in turned into a terror trap.

For a while I comprehended Charley's after-surgery behavior the same way I did his postictal psychosis. I waited for an end day after day, fully expecting his demeanor to change. Then one night reality sank in and I realized Charley was not going to instantly become a nice man. His insanity was capable of keeping him awake for countless days and nights. I knew, though at that time I had not slept for several nights, I was going to fall asleep sometime. I was afraid if I fell asleep Charley might unknowingly murder me.

I cannot explain what it feels like to fear being murdered and at the same time, as a caretaker, feel obligated to take care of an individual who cannot care for themselves. At times I think my soul walked away from my body and watched my life as it was happening. I was exhausted and more worried about how much my children and grandchildren would miss me than I was about living anymore. I no longer prayed for protection. The responsibility for Charley's medical care had been mine. My choices had ultimately caused the terror that was happening in our home. Good intentions or not I had brought whatever happened upon myself. I prayed and asked God to allow me to see my children and grandchildren once more. I wished to give them keepsakes to cherish and remember me by and whisper my good-byes to them within my heart.

In his right mind Charley would never have threatened or tried to intimidate me. Neither of us were in our right mind. I thought of the irony of sacrificing in order to provide the best life I could in spite of Charley's illnesses and my reward was going to be him murdering me and he wouldn't even know what he had done.

I felt sorry for Charley but did not know what to do. Leaving him was not an option. Regardless of the danger he was sick and could not help his actions. Charley was taking medication but was too checked out of reality to remember the dosages. He couldn't prepare meals or fend for himself. He spent every minute on the move lost within a turbulence; sweating, pacing and obsessively speaking his thoughts as he paced more.

I felt a huge responsibility and resolved to do my best to take care of him as long as possible. After several weeks of this nonstop insanity I could not stop crying. One morning Charley threatened me with a knife. I waited until he was napping then I called the medical staff in Dallas and begged for help. I do not remember who I spoke with (more like blubbered to) but told her I was quite sure my husband was going to kill me if he did not get help. She made arrangements to re-admit Charley to the epilepsy clinic at Parkland. Sweet, compassionate, nice lady, whoever you were, thank you. I will always believe you saved my life.

Everything that should have been helpful to our situation created another problem. How on earth was I going to get Charley in the van to take a six hour trip and be readmitted into the hospital? He was convinced he was seeing reality for the first time in his life and everything was fine, except on occasion he thought I probably needed to not breathe anymore. He did not see me cry from his torture even when I cried in front of him and had no clue the stress he was causing or the insanity of his actions. Out of desperation I lied and told him Dr. Diaz-Arrastia wanted to readmit him to the hospital to check for seizures.

Charley had been obsessively putting a metal roof on an old house and was very disappointed I agreed for him to be readmitted to the hospital. After begging for a day I finally convinced him to comply with the doctor's wishes. He cried and cried as we prepared to return to Dallas because he had no clue his behavior was unacceptable. At that time he was more obsessed on fixing that roof than he was on seeing reality or paying me back for his misery. This new obsession calmed his demeanor quite a bit. I was afraid after the roof was finished it would only be a matter of time before the reality he conjured up reached a more violent level than I could wiggle out of.

Though Charley's intimidating behavior somewhat receded while working on the roof his actions became more bizarre every day. When I walked toward him he quickly and dramatically backed away as if I had some deathly, contagious disease. What the hell? His suddenly backing away startled me and when I asked what he was doing he sharply and repetitively said, "Nothing, ma'am, nothing ma'am, nothing ma'am," as he abruptly marched backwards. There was no question; we had to go back to Dallas.

The return trip was one of the saddest experiences I have ever endured. We both cried most of the way. Charley felt trapped and cried because he was obsessing, not understanding why he had to go back in the hospital. His demeanor was that of a child who was being punished for a wrong he did not commit.

He kept saying, "I am not having seizures so why do I have to go back?"

I cried because I did understand why he had to return to the hospital. My heart struggled with the love I felt for Charley and the responsibility I carried for his well-being as an individual. It was so sad that such a good man had to endure the heartache created by unfair medical circumstances and not even know what the hell was happening.

"God help us, do whatever you can." I prayed as we made our way back to the epilepsy unit, "Lord, if we don't stop this blubbering and get it together before arriving at the hospital someone will surely admit us both to the funny farm, lock the doors and throw away the key."

I was so damn tired.

We arrived at the hospital with puffy eyes and tear stained faces. Charley was admitted to the epilepsy unit and monitors were hooked up to him. He never had a seizure but was observed obsessively arguing with me. I tried to explain his behavior to the doctors but was never given the opportunity to speak to them alone. Since Charley was not working on the roof his mind had reverted back to I see reality mode and he was not happy with me. He told me I should be the one in that hospital bed being checked for mental problems. He was fine and could prove it because he saw reality.

I was exhausted and frustrated. I had heard I see reality at least eight billion times and was sick to death of the phrase. Nothing Charley saw at this time was reality, nothing. I wished I could write I see reality on a baseball bat and knock him upside the head with the bat. Though my frustration caused me to think of a million ways to shove I see reality up every orifice on my husband's body, he never knew it. I tried to not let my frustration override my empathy for Charley's needs. Many times I left the hospital room cursing under my breath. Then I breathed deeply, composed myself, and returned to my husband's side to endure another onslaught of "I see reality."

One morning a doctor came into the room and visited. I briefly explained the insanity we were enduring without talking about the intimidating behavior with knives in front of Charley. There was no reason to upset him further. The doctor understood the behavior was inappropriate and stated, "This is when the spouse usually leaves." Immediately after the doctor left the room Charley stated, "I knew it, I knew I saw reality." The doctor's words, to Charley, meant HE should leave me because he was the mistreated spouse. He did not understand the doctor meant most spouses in MY position would leave their partners due to their extreme behavior. I ran and found the doctor and asked him to return to the room and explain the meaning of his statement. Even with the doctor's explanation firmly in place the reality Charley saw was that he was normal and I was crazy and he should leave me. I got no mercy.

At our request Charley was referred to the mental health clinic in Dallas. We thought since their doctors had dealt with people who had undergone brain surgery Charley would get better care with them than the mental health doctor in Amarillo. They prescribed a mood stabilizer that slowed down Charley's behavior but did not stop it.

One morning Charley was checked out of reality and started playing with a knife, acting like he was cleaning his fingernails with it and staring at me with his crazy intimidating look. I realized I could not take him to Dallas every time his behavior went awry. I called Dr. Nguyen, the mental health doctor at the Veteran's Hospital in Amarillo, and she told me to bring him to her office immediately.

Dr. Nguyen asked Charley if he was trying to intimidate me with a knife. He admitted to the act but did not think anything of it because he never really meant to use the knife. She told Charley he could no longer take out his anger on me. Dr. Nguyen said when he became aggravated or felt out of control to write down his thoughts and feelings and share what he had written with her during his next visit. Charley obsessively argued and tried in every way to prove he had no mental problems; thus showing Dr. Nguyen he did, indeed, have mental problems. Dr. Nguyen prescribed an anti-psychotic medication; something I think should have been done by the mental health doctor's in Dallas and might have been prescribed if we had continued our consultations with them. The medication stopped the extreme episodes of intimidation but did not help with obsessive and compulsive behavior. The anti-psychotic medications laid something down in Charley's mind and took a lot of him away. One part of him resented me greatly for having to take those medicines but somewhere deep within him another part loved and trusted me because he took the medications faithfully. Charley never physically laid a hand on me after surgery but he sure scared me.

On one of Charley's worse days I tried to explain to him that maybe some of his actions and reactions were not normal due to his brain needing time to heal. He construed my words as telling him he was insane and unable to maintain. I found a note written during that episode where he states, "This has been a very hard day to keep my physical ability of dangerous being to exist. Seems as if when the noticing of my writing appears the atmosphere seems to improve (maybe I should write all the time). I really upset her again today by using the manners I was taught as a child. Things like saying ma'am - backing out of way of events, happenings, etc."

It breaks my heart that I was enemy no matter my efforts. I remember that day because he was sneering at me as if writing was getting me back. I was always happy to see him release his feelings on paper. The atmosphere calmed when he wrote, but that was not often.

After a few weeks of taking the anti-psychotic medication Charley's intimidating behavior stopped. He still survived within a turbulence and was compulsive and obsessive but usually when the noise of the jet engines was surrounding him he ventured to his shop or found a project to keep busy. As time passed he maintained at a pretty stable level as long as he had something to keep him occupied. We plodded through these trying times as we had always muddled along, sometimes crying, astounded and emotionally drained. Each of our sanity levels were pushed beyond the maximum limit. We endured and did our best to rock along and find a comfortable niche we could fit in together.

Dr. Mickey told us it would take two years for Charley's brain to completely heal from the surgery. On the second anniversary of brain surgery I brought home a cake with the words "congratulations on your new brain" written on it (I had to tell the lady at the bakery the words I wanted written on the cake a dozen times). I bought Charley a new straw hat to wear when he was outside to protect his healed brain from too much sun. We had a party with our grandchildren and celebrated our unusual anniversary and looked forward to the progress his brain, and our life, would surely make throughout the next years.

Seventy days later my Charley died.

When Hospice stepped into our life we knew death was near. Wherever Charley went I trailed behind like a lost puppy, unable to come to grips with the reality of my husband's impending death. I could not face knowing that his next journey was going to be without me. One evening Charley sat on the couch in our living room. Our roles had reversed. I was sitting on the floor at his feet, tying my entire being to the earth, letting the natural flow of the world enter my system to stay calm and endure the physical pain my broken heart was feeling. The last weeks of his life Charley comforted and kept watch over me as his soul slowly slipped away and my soul endured the horrible pain of knowing I was losing him. Through unstoppable tears, as Charley lovingly ran his fingers through my hair and consoled me, I jokingly told him that a million times I had wished to kill him, but I never, ever, ever, ever really wanted him to die.

I do not know what the future may have been if Charley had survived. After surgery, on good days, his mental capacities stayed on a somewhat even keel. On bad days I feared the inability of keeping him mentally stable. Charley's fortitude can serve as an example to others facing the challenges that epilepsy, seizures, psychosis and brain surgery create.

The ability to draw a precise map with all the trails brain surgery will lead others down would be a miracle. No matter how we preplan our journeys some unexpected events will cause detours. Charley's brain surgery was another way to fight epilepsy and prove seizures would never win. If our story inspires anyone to fight a little harder or helps them persevere then Charley and I are still doing our part to battle epilepsy and make sure seizures never win. Hold to your course if you are on the road to eliminating seizures by having brain surgery. In spite of the difficulties the road is well worth traveling.

Chapter 18

Healing, Progression and Sanity after Surgery

I want to share many of the positive aspects of life after surgery. I hope to speak to individuals and couples faced with the prospect of having brain surgery to eliminate seizures. The purpose of this book is not to panic and scare anyone out of having brain surgery by presenting our frightening insanity. We may never know the reasons for Charley's after-surgery behaviors. Dr. Mickey said our circumstances were not common and he speaks the truth. I write about our experiences, both good and bad, to help those who have less severe cases of epilepsy and also to reach the few people who may find themselves living with extreme circumstances.

To anyone contemplating surgery I am very sorry for the fear you are feeling. Fear and indecision are horrible emotions to have ruling your life. We tearfully fought through many doubts and maybes before surgery as we wished for a light at the end of the tunnel. None of the maybes I imagined came true, though some of my doubts did haunt me. Overall the entire experience was completely different than I imagined.

This chapter contains less words than the previous chapter but that is not because the negative circumstances outweighed the positive aspects of our after-surgery life. Charley's irrational behavior lasted only a few months and was over. He became a new man. When he leveled mentally and physically he was busy every day working on projects he could never have undertaken prior to surgery.

Charley lived a little more than two years after surgery. It took about three months after surgery for him to get well enough to start on the projects he finished before he died. His health began to rapidly decline in October of 2005 and he did not work much after. He accomplished an amazing amount of work within a span of about fourteen months. If he were alive now there would not be enough pages to detail everything he would have completed or all the positive aspects of his life.

After surgery Charley and I rocked along in the best way two people who have more love for each other than sense can rock along. When the anti-psychotic medication kicked in we began living within a new level of life. Not one day was our life what most people would consider normal but our life had never been normal so that was nothing new.

When Charley's mentality leveled out and he was not constantly trying to survive within the turbulence of jet engines life was pretty darn good for him. My soul slowly accepted the fact that I no longer had to faithfully protect him. I gradually struggled through retraining my innermost self by forcing myself to give Charley space and speaking aloud, "Stop looking for him; he is never going to have another seizure." I adjusted to the fact (never fully, but the best I could) that I no longer had to continually worry about a seizure. Life slowly became much better for me.

I thanked God daily for answering our prayers and granting us a seizure-free life. Our family and I had spread the word to everyone for prayers regarding Charley's healing. I felt that was enough to ask of my friends and family and did not accurately know how to share with anyone my imperfections that were caused by living with Charley's epilepsy. I tearfully prayed alone for God to help and heal me.

As time passed and the Lord guided us through our healing we began to communicate and enjoy each other's company. Some days we talked for hours. Before surgery Charley could not communicate. My words must have all sounded the same when he was constantly fighting seizures. After surgery he listened and understood and we had many wonderful, laughter filled conversations that never could have occurred without surgery. We enjoyed our time talking about Charley's new realizations. Our morning conversations are some of my most tender memories. To some people regular conversation is not something treasured but when you live in the world of seizures many everyday events that are taken for granted by others are not a part of life. Relaxed conversation was one of those things.

One of the most exciting and wonderful events after surgery was Charley passing the driver's exam and being reissued a driver's license.

I can still see the smug smile on his face when he realized he would no longer be dependent on others for transportation. Charley could go anywhere he wanted and I encouraged him to enjoy his new freedom.

The first Christmas after regaining his driving privileges I gave Charley one-hundred dollars for a present. I told him to go buy anything he wanted. He was excited and overwhelmed. Charley said he was going to Amarillo which is about forty miles from our home. I was apprehensive about his traveling alone but could not wait to see the fruits of his shopping adventure. He was gone for several hours while I imagined him browsing at every store. Charley returned home and bustled into the front door smiling the biggest smile I have ever seen.

"What did you buy?" I anxiously asked as I ran to the door to hug him and make sure he was still in one piece.

Charley said, "Nothing. I was so damn excited to be driving around that far from home I never did get out anywhere to shop. I just drove around."

I was sitting at home imagining unloading his bounty while he was driving around like a kid enjoying his first bumper car experience at the fair! I sat on the couch and laughed so hard I had tears running down my face.

When I composed myself I said, "Charley, you could have bought nothing here!"

Then we both laughed until we cried. Isn't that great? The best gifts surgery gave to Charley no amount of money could purchase; answered prayers, freedom, the ability to work, the privilege of driving, enjoying his independence, communication, renewed confidence, clear thoughts, smiles and new adventures. These things Charley deserved and so enjoyed when he could process the world around him. The ability to drive a vehicle is taken for granted by many people. For Charley and I the loss of his driving privileges was huge but we did not quit fighting seizures and we won. If you ever quit fighting seizures you will not win. Brain surgery? Yes, have the surgery.

One thing that was very hard for me after Charley's surgery was to accept the fact that we could no longer work together. Obsessive thought patterns somewhat ruled his behavior and if I tried to help him on projects I was an interruption, not a helper. I had to respect the brain work he did to keep his thoughts straight and leave him alone when he was trying to complete a project. Giving Charley space was very difficult but I did my best. I slowly regained some of my individuality that was lost over the years due to the responsibility of keeping him safe. Learning to build and accept healthy separation was completely foreign but a good thing for us.

Charley managed to single-handedly accomplish a mind boggling amount of work that he never would have been able to do had he been having seizures. He put a metal roof on an old house we owned. We could not afford to buy new metal so he did a lot of extra work in cutting rusty corrugated metal to length and patching it. Charley did a fine job and the roof still does not leak. The task may sound simple for anyone who never lived with seizures but for Charley it was one he could not have attempted before surgery. It would have been unsafe for him to climb the ladder, stand on the roof or use the saw for cutting the metal. His mind was so weak by the time of surgery he had no energy or ability to plan any job. After surgery Charley tackled that roof until it was completed. He had a small window of energy, only four to five hours before he was too tired to continue but seizures were not the culprit keeping him from being productive. After finishing that job Charley then put a new metal roof on two other storage buildings.

The next project Charley tackled was to re-trim our house. He had never been happy with the trim we used when we built the house. I did not want to redo the trim but he insisted we needed to update and was right. We set up scaffolding and he proceeded to tear off every piece of corner and window trim on the first and second floors. I was conditioned to losing tomorrows due to seizures so I was apprehensive as I pictured every critter in the Texas Panhandle crawling in where the trim had been. Seizures were no longer stealing our time. Charley was unable to work long hours but worked on that trim every day until the job was complete and skillfully done. Perhaps that sounds like an everyday job to some but before surgery the degree of Charley's seizures left a very skilled carpenter with the desire to work but no ability. He climbed up and down, stood on the top platform, and leaned over scaffolding that was twenty feet tall. Before surgery he sat seizure stunned in a worn recliner, too sick to use his tools. He was barely able to comprehend what was on the television he watched just to keep from going completely crazy. Did the surgery help? You bet, the surgery helped Charley – a lot!

After the trim was finished we caulked and painted our house. I did help with this task though I had to learn to maintain a healthy distance and allow Charley's thoughts to flow without interruption. We both painted the trim and I did my best not to interrupt his thought patterns. I caught myself constantly observing Charley and repeatedly whispered to my soul, "Stop watching him. He is never going to have another seizure."

Next Charley installed rain gutter on the house. He had to concentrate very hard to accomplish this. I realized he needed his thoughts uninterrupted more than my help. He happily climbed scaffolding day after day to install rain gutter on the first and second floors. No one could have done a more professional job. I did not have to worry for one second that Charley might seizure and fall. Keeping a distance was a struggle but I was slowly accepting that I could leave him alone.

Charley completed many other tasks but the last project was building our front porch. We had most of the materials stockpiled in garages. He realized the porch could be built with a minimal amount of expense and immediately went to work. While Charley built the porch we were only a window apart. I watched him through the study window while I sat at my computer writing this book. I typed away while Charley leveled dirt, dug postholes, mixed and poured cement, and set the posts. Letting him work alone was difficult but I managed, though I did wiggle in and help some. Charley built the frame, put the floor on, set rafters, laid plywood on the roof and metal on top of that. "Don't forget to buy the rain gutter, Lo." he told me as I was leaving to purchase supplies. Charley installed rain gutter and painted the underside of the plywood and within a couple of months was finished with a beautiful porch that spans the entire front of the house. The porch was the last project needed to complete the construction of our home that we started building in 1998. We both felt a great sense of accomplishment as we giggled about memories created building our largest, and most beautiful, construction project. We spent wonderful summer mornings on that porch drinking coffee and visiting and many evenings laughing and reminiscing surrounded by our loving family.

The projects Charley completed are only one positive outcome of his undergoing surgery. Even when obsessing and driving me crazy he was busy which is a great improvement over living in a daze due to seizures. I cannot express all the immense ways brain surgery helped my husband.

It is irrational to advise anyone contemplating brain surgery to feel no fear. There are many reasons to be afraid. If you elect for surgery try to build strength from the hope you must be seeking. Not one thing I say or anything you imagine will prepare you for the specific outcome of your surgery. If you are hoping to eliminate seizures by electing for brain surgery I can positively say everything we went through after surgery was worth regaining a large part of our life. Charley fought having seizures for over twenty years with every bit of strength his mind could muster and when that strength gave out he fought having seizures by having brain surgery. It took a while, but many good things came about because of Charley's decision. Don't wait until clusters of seizures are making you psychotic to seek brain surgery. Take your life away from epilepsy as soon as possible.

Chapter 19
Agreements of Trust

If you are having brain surgery there are a million questions in your mind. Being prepared for every occurrence during and after surgery is impossible. I have thought about every aspect of Charley's after-surgery behaviors and what we could have done to make our life easier. Based upon the assertion that trust is the most important aspect of any relationship I have written this chapter.

I never could have anticipated the different person Charley's surgery made of him. I sure wasn't prepared to be the cause of so many problems because of my past conditioning. I was very over-protective and Charley no longer needed protecting. Another aspect neither of us was prepared for was his irrational behavior. I highly recommend to anyone who is preparing for brain surgery to seek counseling whether you are alone or a couple. The staff in Dallas required Charley to have a mental health doctor but I had no help and we had no help as a couple. Find a counselor for everyone involved to speak to before and after the surgery. It may take some research but find a doctor who can prepare everyone for dealing with the changes surgery will create.

If you are the caretaker of a person who has seizures you will not easily adjust to a new life without seizures dictating your every move. My mind knew Charley was not going to seizure but my instincts told me to jump every time he moaned or looked like he might fall. Living with a seizure-free Charley was harder for a while than living with him when he had seizures. I knew the routine before surgery and I was lost afterward.

One idea that may help with the trying situations that arise after surgery is for the person being operated on and their primary caregiver to sign an Agreement of Trust before surgery. An agreement on paper between both parties to remind them of their primary duties during the healing process would be a handy tool. I have never seen an Agreement of Trust so I have written one for each person involved in the surgery. The agreements are at the end of this chapter. After Charley's surgery

I wished a billion times for something to show him that might break through his fog. I wanted a paper that said, "you trusted me before this damn surgery . . . you have to trust me now." I also wished for a way to help Charley understand that I was going through a personal brain trauma of my own as I dealt with all of my mental adjustments.

I had nothing to fall back on to help my husband keep in perspective that his brain needed to heal before his life would be normal. I could have placed an Agreement of Trust in his hands and told him he had read and signed it before surgery. A firm explanation that we knew and agreed before surgery there were going to be adjustments would have helped our situation. Placing something in his hands that reminded him of the trust he felt for me might have calmed Charley during the hard times. Tearing the paperwork to shreds would have been better than taking his frustrations out on me. Come to think of it making several copies of the agreement might not be a bad idea.

There were times Charley placing an Agreement of Trust that I had signed into my hands and reminding me to abide by my commitments would have helped him. Sometimes I was impatient when he had no clue what needs I had. Other times I was irritatingly over-protective and failed to respect Charley's new life. It would have been nice to have something we could both grasp to remind us of our mutual trust when we did not know how to emotionally deal with our circumstances.

Charley's medical staff prepared us the best they could for the outcome of his surgery. Unless a person has had brain surgery or lived with someone after surgery there is no way to know the future circumstances. We were warned of severe headaches, scars, potential infections, short term memory loss and how long it would take for a brain to fully heal. Every after-surgery minute is difficult for a while. You must prepare yourself every way possible. Use this Agreement of Trust as an example then sit down together and outline what changes you expect to come about through surgery and make your own. Do not go into surgery with blinders on and not be prepared for a time of healing and change afterward. Brain surgery requires a lot of patience and understanding from both sides.

Agreement of Trust
I Am Having Surgery

I am going to have brain surgery and need my partner to help me through. Thank you for being with me and making this as comfortable as possible for both of us. I am signing this agreement for you to show me during rough moments of my healing.

I understand after surgery I must allow myself time to heal and my thoughts and actions may not always be rational. I will depend on you more than I am accustomed to as you comfort me. I may become depressed and will have a mental health doctor after surgery. I understand the most important element of our relationship is trust and I do trust you. After my initial healing I will participate in and enjoy life.

I want to declare my full trust in you before surgery because I know you always have my best interests at heart. I understand after surgery you will present this agreement to me if I need to be reminded of who always protects and takes care of me.

We are stepping into the unknown together and this surgery will be difficult for you. I will do my best to allow myself to heal as you help me.

I understand you will present this agreement to me if you feel I am being impatient or causing you to be uncomfortable or unhappy.

_____

Signature of Surgery Patient

Agreement of Trust
I am Going Through Surgery
With You

I am going to be your partner and caretaker throughout your brain surgery and recovery. Thank you for allowing me to be with you during this time. I want to make this surgery as comfortable as possible. I am signing this agreement so you can show it to me during rough moments of your healing and remind me that we both knew this was not going to be easy.

I understand after the surgery I must allow you to rest, recover and heal. Your thoughts may not always be rational and I will help you through those times. I will comfort you and be dependable in helping with your needs. If either of our actions deem it necessary we will immediately see the mental health doctor.

I will always be truthful. I also understand after your initial healing you will participate in and enjoy life.

Recovery may be difficult. I will do my best to be a good caretaker as I stay calm and rational and allow you the time to heal. I cherish the trust you place in me. I will always have your best interests at heart.

I understand you will present this agreement to me if you feel I am being impatient or making you uncomfortable or unhappy.

_____

Signature of Caretaker/Parent/Spouse/Partner

Life
After
Surgery

Chapter 20

Be Ready to Encounter a New World

Before Charley's surgery if I had been given warning that part of his healing process would result in an unintentional destructive nature I could have prevented damage to our possessions. Anyone considering brain surgery should be forewarned that their nature may change for a while after surgery. Charley's behavior differences did not last forever but with the initial trauma many different personality characteristics surfaced. The longer he healed the better these characteristics became and his personality smoothed out. Even the overpowering obsessive behavior became something we both learned to manage and often found humorous.

The obsessive behavior slowly diminished but did not ever completely stop. Charley's two dominant obsessions were pleasing me and fixing everything we owned that he thought needed maintenance. With his brain working on low capacity most of what he attempted to repair was torn to pieces. His true motive behind everything he did was pleasing me. Praising Charley's work was very important to his well-being. He was crushed when he thought I was unhappy. However, it was very difficult to look at an expensive piece of equipment he ruined and not express my unhappiness about the destruction. When I understood how disheartened he became over my displeasure I learned to conceal my feelings.

Charley told me one day he was going to fix the cable that opened the hood on our car. I was afraid he might carry the thought into an obsession so I went to the car and opened the hood to see if the cable was broken. It worked fine and I took Charley to the car and showed him. I made him pull the cable handle and open the hood several times thinking surely if he saw there was nothing wrong he would not attempt to fix it. He promised to leave the car alone but the obsessive thought that the cable was broken overrode his promise.

I ran some errands and returned home after a few hours. When I arrived home the doomed car was in front of the shop. I stepped out of my car and slowly made my way to where Charley was unknowingly lying in the dirt working on the car. I took a deep breath and had some much needed self-talk.

Charley had managed to pull the cable from under the dash until it was stretched several feet lying on the ground past the rear wheel of the car. Yet; that cable was still attached under the hood.

He said, "I am fixing the car."

I did not show disappointment or anger toward him. When confronted with an upsetting situation I trained myself to repeat back to Charley whatever he said.

I said to him, "You sure are fixing the car." I gave him a kiss on the cheek and went into the house before my willpower crumbled and I verbalized my thoughts.

When Charley did mechanical work his mind entered into a running obsession. He shut out everything and tore stuff to pieces thinking he was making a repair. If the rest of the car had to be thrown into the trash pile he was going to repair that cable. It was hard to leave him alone destroying our car but I did. I worked on a chapter in this book because I knew interrupting in the middle of an obsession would cause Charley more distress than the car being torn to pieces was causing me.

When our son, Alan, arrived home from work that evening Charley had pulled the cable from under the dash to the back bumper of the car and still not opened the hood. To Charley the sensible thing to do was remove the front bumper, headlights, grill, running lights, radiator and any other parts of the car he could unbolt. He obsessively tore the car to pieces because he could not get the hood open and fix a cable that a wrinkle in his brain decided was broken.

When Alan arrived I was outside silently walking in circles around the haphazardly scattered pile of car parts Charley's obsession had produced. Alan understood that his dad was healing from surgery and would never have been unpleasant.

Alan told Charley, "It is alright, dad, I can fix this in no time." and within a few seconds he opened the hood.

I went into the house because I could not contain my laughter over the look on Alan's face. Seeing him mirror me, sucking in his breath and stopping himself from saying anything negative to Charley was hilarious. Shortly afterward Alan followed and sat in the room with me. I could not contain my laughter. Alan was so aggravated. He described the frustrating moments we endured after Charley's surgery as "hang on just a minute while I go around the corner and scream into a bag." It felt so good to have someone share my frustration.

I wiped tears of laughter out of my eyes and Alan said, "Mom, I wish you would make him leave stuff alone until I get home." I could only look at my exasperated son and laugh. Within a few seconds we looked out of the window and saw Charley rapidly walking toward the house. Alan masked his frustration and I quickly composed myself. When Charley came in the house and discovered us sitting together in the study we were calm and collected.

Alan nonchalantly said, "Dad, I will be back out in a minute and help with the car." Charley quickly walked out of the door and headed toward his scattered pile of car.

After I composed myself I asked Alan, "Do you remember when you were a child what your dad used to say when he came home to bicycle parts and pieces strewn all over the yard?"

I told Alan when he and his brother, Chaeton, were young and tried to fix their bicycles Charley always came to me and said, "I wish you would make them leave stuff alone until I get home!" I giggled and explained to Alan that the parent-child roles had switched. Now his dad was in distress and Alan the one expected to fix something that should not have been torn up. We both laughed as I told him at this rate my senility should kick in and I would be next in line for him to switch roles with. He shook his head and went outside to repair the car.

A few days later Charley repaired our riding lawn mower. That time, though Alan tried while I giggled at his masked frustration, the damage to the mower could not be fixed. Nuts, bolts, pulleys, both blades and other parts to the mower were slung all over the yard when Charley started the mower and engaged the blades after making his repairs. I forbid him to do any more mechanical work as nicely as I could. I praised his carpentry skills and asked him to please concentrate on building, refinishing furniture and fixing our house. He conceded and we did not have any more obsessive incidences with mechanical items.

Another changed personality characteristic Charley adjusted to after surgery was the inability to complete crossword puzzles. Prior to surgery his vocabulary was huge and crossword puzzles were one of his favorite pastimes. After surgery though he knew what the questions meant he could not formulate the correct words for the answers. Specific details and one word answers baffled him. Charley expressed his disappointment about the inability to finish crossword puzzles to our family but no one understood. They had never been interested in working crossword puzzles so they did not empathize. The inability to work the puzzles surprised Charley and was frustrating but he did not give up. Every evening he worked on crossword puzzles rebuilding his word dictionary.

A funny personality characteristic popped up at the same time Charley was trying to grasp and put words to meanings. He began to have what we called "word of the day" occurrences. His brain picked a word and everything was described by that word. One word was enhancing and everything was enhancing. He said, "Thank you for breakfast, it was very enhancing" And, "It sure is enhancing to be married to you." Or, "I think it would be enhancing to go outside." Statements such as, "The car is sure enhancing today." were said every day. We both became so tickled about his "word of the day" we could hardly contain our laughter. He had no control over the word his brain grasped and no idea when his brain would let the word go. No matter how hard he tried not to speak the word it involuntarily described everything. I cannot specifically remember any other words that overtook Charley's speech but there were others but none so much as enhancing. Some wrinkle in his brain frequently latched on to the word enhancing and he stated the word repeatedly until his brain healed enough to release that habit.

If you live with, or are taking care of a person that has had brain surgery expect some changed personality characteristics. When their pain diminishes enough to allow healing to progress they become more active but are not well enough to be accountable for many of their behaviors. Be kind, they cannot control their flaws. If they obsess they obsess. If they tear things up then things are torn up. If they speak inappropriately so be it. A person healing from brain surgery should not be degraded, overly corrected, treated harshly or a victim of anger.

I will be the first to say that constantly being patient and kind is a huge goal to set and impossible to accomplish. I was not perfect when dealing with Charley's after-surgery personality characteristics. It is very difficult to leave the house in the morning and drive past your undamaged vehicle and come home to a pile of bolts and pieces and not blow your stack. I thought it a good sign that Charley felt well enough to work until I came home to a heap of rubbish that was a car and dodged lawn mower parts flying all over our front yard. For more than a year after surgery Charley's mind trapped little things and created big things from them. I knew there would be changes but I was not prepared and had no idea how to deal with them.

I was lucky to have lived with Charley's pre-surgery psychotic behavior because it prepared me for the unknown and taught me to be observant and patient. I giggled about Charley's bizarre behavior rather than becoming upset. It was an easier journey when I looked for humor rather than allowing myself to be blinded by frustration.

If you are associated with a person who has brain surgery be observant during the healing process and brace yourself for unexpected personality changes. Build strength and understanding from the knowledge that one person's inability to control their actions does not equal another person's unwillingness to control their reactions.

Chapter 21

Thinking Backwards and Upside Down

When I attempt to explain Charley's after-surgery behaviors and thought patterns most people do not comprehend how unique they were. In an attempt to keep Charley busy with construction projects I had him build a set of shelves in a shed we owned so we could organize. I placed various items in numbered tubs. He placed the tubs on the shelves beginning with the number one. His tub organization showed me how his brain was processing several months after surgery. Rather than starting the number 1 tub on the left hand side of the shelves he went to the far right corner of the room and placed the number 1 tub on the top right-hand corner of the shelf. Then tub 2 was to the left then tub 3. He then placed tubs 4, 5 and 6 right to left on the second shelf. Then tubs 7, 8 and 9 right to left on the third shelf and tubs 10, 11 and 12 were below that from right to left and so on. Charley could have placed the tubs in numeric order from left to right, with tubs 1 through 9 on the top shelf, then 10 through 18 on the next shelf and tubs 19 through 27 on the third shelf and tubs 22 through 30 on the next shelves but he didn't.

The order of the tubs was placed from right to left because that is how his brain worked without a left temporal lobe. He did not place the tubs left to right as his brain was trained to do before surgery. With no left temporal lobe he placed them in groups of three with the numeric order of the tubs backwards (right to left). I learned that Charley's brain grouped data in small manageable sets and no longer processed from the left to the right.

After completing the job Charley asked for my final approval. A minute of blank staring helped me understand what he had done and slowly comprehend the bizarre order of the tubs. The puzzled look on my face and extended period of silence made Charley realize the tubs' order was bizarre.

He laughed and said, "What in the hell have I done? Lo, I just realized I put these tubs up wrong. Give me a few minutes and I will fix them."

"No, no, no, Charley." I told him as I giggled and shook my head, "Leave the tubs just like that. Don't you see what you did? You made a map of how your brain is processing at this stage of your healing. I like the tubs. It is completely you."

My brain could not instantly take me to any one of those tubs without having to stop, look and stare at the numbers in order to find the correct one. I had to practically stand on my head to find the tubs that were on the lower shelves. As I became oriented to the system I giggled thinking, "Isn't this funny, here I am forcing myself to think like Charley, right to left, backwards and upside down!"

The occasional work my brain did to find the tubs as Charley placed them did not compare to the constant work his brain had to do in order to survive without a left temporal lobe. I looked at those tubs when I was frustrated with my husband and reminded myself to be patient. This was proof that his brain just did not work like most brains and a great reminder that my heart needed to work harder than most in order to establish a sense of balance within our life.

Chapter 22
Who Says the Mind is Kind?

Throughout my life I have heard the statement, "The mind is kind." I often wondered what fool thought up that analogy when I was dragging my husband around like a limp bag of potatoes after he had a seizure. Charley's mind sometimes produced weeks of erratic behavior between episodes of tonic-clonic seizures. If I could not immediately respond to those seizures he wet the bed, bit his tongue, slobbered everywhere and sometimes fell resulting in black eyes and bruises. I had a lot of words to describe Charley's mind, but kind was never one of them. However; after witnessing the many new processes brain surgery brought about I did conclude that the mind is amazing.

A few months after surgery Charley's mind began processing memories differently. For the first time in his life his brain began to process feelings associated with memories that must have been buried somewhere within his mind. Charley remembered details of experiences but unbeknownst to him memories and feelings lived as two separate beings within him. In other words, he was like a person watching television in regard to life experiences. He saw the picture but his feelings were not connected to the memories. Before brain surgery he lived life as it happened, saw events occur and created memories. But, Charley was detached from the normal feelings that he should have felt at the time events occurred and the memories associated with the events were created. After surgery he felt feelings he never knew existed that were tied to events that had unfolded throughout his life. It was not unusual to find Charley crying or hear him crack up laughing when new memories surfaced and he experienced the feelings associated with those memories for the first time.

We talked for hours about Charley's memories and escaping feelings. I was captivated and loved sharing his newly discovered feelings. I could tell by looking in his eyes that he was replaying within his mind life events that he had never faced or understood.

When the channel to his emotions unlocked he had to face the fact that his conclusions and reactions to many previous events had been wrong. He reflected on his first marriage and no longer blamed his ex-wife for divorcing him as he had always done. He understood her decision and felt very bad for the years he had ruthlessly blamed her for their problems.

In 2002 Charley and I adopted our grandson, Eddie, which was a very hard decision. We knew we were doing the right thing for Eddie but the adoption was a very difficult for Charley. He was eleven years older than me and knew if my health deteriorated he could not raise a child alone. Prior to surgery he tried in a million different ways to accept Ed but could not. Charley was very happy when the surgery somehow helped him to accept Eddie as his son and a permanent part of our life. When Charley regained his driving privileges he loaded Eddie in the car almost every day and took him to a small country store a mile from our home for a snow cone and a round of gossip with the old men who sat and visited at a small table in the store. During the summers Charley and Eddie spent hours together in our above-ground swimming pool playing like two children who had each happily found a new best friend.

Feelings! After surgery Charley experienced feelings that led to a lot of self-awareness and forgiveness within his heart that we both needed. He was aware that I never had given up on him and deeply loved me for my devotion.

Charley told our daughter Katie that he knew life had not been easy because of him and assured her those days were finished. Katie cannot talk of that moment without crying. Her childhood was riddled with insanity and adulthood haunted by the anger Charley's psychosis created within her heart. As an adult Kate unselfishly helped us in spite of the damage to her soul living with Charley's psychosis had inflicted. For all of her life Katie had needed her damaged feelings validated by her dad so her wounded heart could heal. Charley's having brain surgery enabled him to help his daughter heal and love him in a way she never could. This was a gift no words can adequately express.

Charley looked back at his callous behavior toward our children during their childhood. There were many events he could not remember but he realized his actions were harsh. He felt nothing ever said could possibly make up for his lack of understanding of their needs as children. He tried to emotionally move beyond the disappointment he felt in himself for not being a more loving and gentle father.

It has been said the mind is kind because it does not let you remember events that are too traumatic. How kind is a mind that allows a person to have memories but disallows them to have feelings? When Charley's headaches subsided after brain surgery the floodgates in his mind were opened. He was a man who had lived all of his life overwhelmed by unexplained resentment and unanswered questions. As feelings surfaced and he dealt with them he slowly became a man of self-understanding.

Sometimes Charley announced, "No wonder," as he told me about circumstances he lived as a child and how it felt to tie his present feelings to that situation. He loved exploring within his mind, conjuring up old situations and reliving them with the feelings most people would have felt at the time the situation occurred.

Charley looked back, connected past emotions to present actions, and made sense of many events that had pushed him over the edge in the past. Processing feelings helped him find an emotional medium he had never experienced. Before surgery Charley's emotions were extreme; love or hate, violent or calm, angry or happy. When the after-surgery insanity passed he worked to weigh out situations and be more rational with his reactions and conclusions. He asked questions and worked to process and understand different feelings associated with emotional extremes. Charley was never without problems and it took a while to establish a somewhat even keel but he did.

Isn't that just awesome? To think a person could actually survive and prosper and not really know what feelings are and then have a surgery that allowed their brain to locate and process over fifty years worth of them? Charley had the hardest time trying to accurately explain what it felt like to find and feel something within himself that he had never known was absent. He said it was like walking on clouds and not falling through.

It has been said the mind is kind when it blocks our memories but I do not agree. I think Charley's buried feelings and unprocessed emotions had a lot to do with his seizures and psychosis. Could lost feelings associated with memories cause emotional churning until a mind could no longer cope?

Our medical community needs to recognize if a psychotic person they are treating has living memories and dead feelings. I do not know if anything short of having his left temporal lobe removed would have allowed Charley to experience feelings. If that link had been found before unprocessed feelings piled up within his mind maybe he could have been helped in different ways and lived a healthier life.

I fell in love, married, and spent twenty-six out of the fifty-four years I have lived with Charley Jines, a man whose mind tortured him every day until the day he died. I most likely would punch out anyone who ever tried to convince me that the mind is kind.

Chapter 23

I Thought Dreams Were Things People Wanted

The psychosis medication slowly calmed Charley's demeanor and after several months we began living a fairly normal life. Then, though he seemed to be resting well and enjoying life a bit more each day, he began to intentionally not sleep. I was puzzled as to why Charley was forcing himself to stay awake when he knew his brain needed rest. On some occasions he went to bed and awoke in the middle of the night and stayed awake in the living room until daylight.

One morning I discovered a very distressed Charley sitting in the living room on our rock fireplace hearth. I knew he had not slept and was afraid he might become depressed or have a headache if he became too tired. I sat down beside him and rubbed his neck and shoulders and asked him to please go back to bed and rest.

"I can't." he tiredly said as he lovingly leaned his body against mine, "I'm seeing stuff in my head when I sleep."

After brain surgery a person goes through many changes. All their caretaker can do is be loving and supportive as they sit on the sidelines and hope for understandable explanations. I always tried to formulate an answer to Charley's troubles to save him from having to explain distressing situations. I processed his words, but could not imagine what he was talking about. Charley felt he had put me through enough and was having a hard time expressing his latest flaw. I realized he had been obsessing over fixing the problem during the nights while he sat alone.

"You are going to have to explain what is going on." I said. "I can't help you if I don't understand."

He stared at me for quite a while as he tried to find different words and then he said, "I am seeing stuff in my head when I sleep."

Well, that certainly helped I thought to myself.

Charley said, "Last night when I was asleep I saw us walking together through a pasture holding hands. It went away when I woke up."

I realized he was dreaming and thought he was looking for some significance to the dream. I tried to make him feel better by interpreting the dream. I told Charley maybe he dreamed and saw us holding hands because we had held on to each other through our darkest times. I also explained that after going through a traumatic experience, such as brain surgery, it takes a while for our minds to accept the circumstances and allow our thoughts to subconsciously process those events. It became apparent by his confused look my explanations were not making sense.

"Why?" Charley asked. I stared a hole through him as I tried to understand our lack of communication.

I said, "Why what, Charley?"

"Why am I seeing stuff in my head when I sleep and why does what I see go away when I wake up?" he asked.

"Charley, you are dreaming." I told him.

In the most serious tone he said, "What in the hell are you talking about? Dreaming? In my sleep?"

He sat silent for a few moments contemplating my statement and then said, "I thought dreams were things people wanted."

I discovered through a confusing conversation that Charley thought dreams were possessions or wishes people wanted. Dreaming, in his mind, was something you said not something you did. Can you imagine going to square one and trying to explain what a dream is to a fifty-seven year old person who has never dreamed and began dreaming because they had brain surgery? If Charley ever dreamed he sure did not remember. He either had no dream slate or the slate was wiped clean with the removal of his left temporal lobe.

I told Charley that dreams are our subconscious thoughts processing while we sleep and I found myself on the receiving end of a blank stare. I reassured him dreaming was normal and not a flaw he needed to fix.

"I never have." he flatly stated.

I said, "Charley, you aren't having seizures. Your thought processes must be becoming normal as your brain heals. I promise, dreams are normal."

Charley said, "Not in any way, shape or form are they normal. No one looks right even when I can figure out who they are. Stupid things happen that I can't control. Half the time stuff is floating everywhere. I can't feel what I try to touch. And what I hate the most is I see people I never could stand and damn sure don't want to see them while I'm trying to sleep."

Good Grief! Over the years I have done everything to make Charley's hardships easier and he fully expected me to solve this problem.

His next question was, "How do I fix them?"

"Fix what?" I asked as I became more confused by the second.

"Now what in the hell were we just talking about?" Charley strongly asked.

"Well, ummm, well," I stammered, "dreams?"

"Hell, yes, dreams." he said, "How do I fix them?"

My dumbfounded mind was attempting to process the fact that I had been married to a man for over twenty years and had no idea he never dreamed. No wonder he always looked at me like I was an idiot when I told him about my dreams. He had no idea what I was talking about.

As I attempted to come to my senses Charley said, "No, no, now that I think about it I don't want to fix the damn things. I want to stop dreaming completely. How do I do that, Lo?" I was as stunned as Charley was serious. I finally told him there is no way to stop our dreams and explained when we go into a deep sleep our sub-conscious thoughts take over our brains and we dream. Charley walked out of the room and that was the end of the conversation.

The next morning I encountered a very upset Charley in the living room obsessing about dreaming. Right away he said, "You mean to tell me I absolutely cannot make myself stop dreaming?"

"Yes, Charley, that is what I am telling you." I answered.

"Damn." he uttered under his breath, "I can't shut this off somehow?"

"No Charley you cannot shut off your subconscious thoughts." I said. I drank my coffee while he sat silently.

"Ok, I guess I will have to learn how to live with dreaming." he said.

My thoughts began to ease with those words. I hoped my explanations had calmed his mind. Maybe he was beginning to understand what dreams were and why we had them.

His next words were "Lo, how do I make myself dream only what I want to dream about?" Oh, gosh, here we go again.

"Charley . . . honey . . . you can't order yourself to dream a certain dream and that be only what you dream." I stated.

He looked at me for a while and calmly asked, "Why?"

"Charley, subconscious thoughts are not ours to rule." I told him, "Subconscious thoughts are our sleep thoughts. They are what our mind, during our sleep, makes out of events and thoughts we participate in while we are awake." I gently explained.

We comfortably sat in silence as I conjured up images in my mind of all the wheels that were turning in his head.

"Well, I don't like it." Charley said. He did not like dreams but we never had another long discussion about fixing, changing or eliminating them.

Many times Charley told me about his amazing dreams but he never liked dreaming. He expressed his displeasure about dreaming to Denton whom Charley always depended on to fix what I could not. Denton discovered Charley disliked dreams because they were not all good. Charley just wanted everything to be all good.

It took some time for the notion to actually register in my mind and be accepted in my heart that I was married to a man for over twenty years who may never have received a single message from his subconscious thought processes during sleep. I was sorry dreams disturbed Charley but very happy to know another aspect of life was becoming normal because of his choice to have brain surgery. The dreams did not seem normal to Charley but I hoped other processes his brain had not allowed would begin. Maybe in time a peace would sink into his soul that had always been missing. Perhaps he could find the happiness he deserved that had always been so elusive.

I often wondered if psychosis or seizures robbed Charley of his subconscious thoughts. What other normal things had he managed to survive all of life without that the rest of us took for granted? I wonder if he had been in touch with his subconscious thoughts and able to process them in a healthy manner would he have been psychotic? Does one mental inability replace or rob the other mental ability? Did psychosis push his subconscious thought processes aside and create seizures? Or did seizures create the psychosis which in turn took away the ability to normally process subconscious thought?

Brain surgery to eliminate seizures was not an option when Charley was a young man. He often tearfully told me he would never wish it on his worst enemy to suffer and be robbed of their life the way he had been due to seizures. Charley did not have brain surgery only for himself. Being an older man he knew that he was not going to live a long life. His greatest hope was that having surgery would help teach the medical profession something that could be used to help someone else. He wanted to help pave the way for new generations to stop their seizures by having surgery.

Charley had it right. Dreams are things that people want. There are many people in the world not living the life they want because of seizures. If our story inspires others to find the strength to pursue their dreams and live the life they want that would have made my Charley very happy!

Epilepsy Unveiled

Chapter 24
Sifting Through Memories

At times I sit in front of my computer tapping away at the keyboard as memories unfold and words take shape. Other occasions something pulls at my heart but I do not understand what memory is attempting to surface. I cannot visually picture past circumstances well enough to put them on paper. When a past event I cannot identify pulls at my thoughts I take a pen and notepad and sit on the couch and write by hand. Thoughts that surprise me flow from my heart and out the end of my fingertips onto the paper. These are memories kept in my heart yet pushed aside by my mind.

A couple of weeks ago I wrote by hand as feelings flowed. I had no idea what my heart was trying to tell me until the sentences took shape. It is strange to live with memories that you cannot remember. Trauma does that to a brain, makes it forget in order to survive . . . or . . . makes it survive in order to forget.

My friend Kathy is a very loving, smart individual who has graciously consented to helping with my book by proof reading each chapter. She is our local Postmaster and I see her almost every day. Kathy is my someone that is helping me help someone neither of us know yet by encouraging me. Charley and I both knew Kathy and saw her almost every day as we suffered with seizures and he underwent surgery.

I thought the feelings I write about in the next chapter were caused by my grief over Charley's death and insignificant. I talked to Kathy about them and she encouraged me to share the memories. She felt the subject very important and said it did not matter if grief had caused these memories to emerge. I sit tapping on the keyboard again as I use the notes I wrote to express another aspect of living with epilepsy both before and after surgery. These memories were hidden beneath years of unshed tears buried deep within my soul. After reliving them I stopped writing for a couple of weeks in order to work through grief and gather mental strength. They hit hard in the core of my being.

Thus the background to the next chapter.

Epilepsy Unveiled

Chapter 25

I Have Never Seen Myself Have a Seizure

When I took Charley to a doctor, usually, the first question the doctor asked was, "When did you have your last seizure?" Charley jokingly replied, "Hell, I don't know. I am not awake when I have a seizure. Maybe I haven't had any seizures. I have never seen myself have a seizure." Then he asked, "Lo, when did I have my last seizure?"

The doctor usually giggled at Charley's bizarre answers, but I did not. Deep down, I knew my husband's statement held a huge truth about the way he felt toward the role I played in correlation to his seizures. Charley had never seen himself have a seizure.

In his mind I was the person saying he had seizures, taking him to the doctor, and telling him to take medication for a condition he had never seen. I was the only person Charley had to be angry with when he had to surrender his driver's license. I reminded him of what activities might cause seizures and stopped him from participating in activities he wanted to do. I was the person his irrational behavior was blamed on and directed toward. When Charley asked me "Lo, when did I have my last seizure?" those words were not said in trust and faith. They were spoken by a non-believer and a bystander to his own illness; a stranger who lived in the same house with me for years yet a person who never witnessed himself having a seizure . . . so perhaps all this stuff about having seizures was not real.

In Charley's mind his illness was not as serious as Lola made it out to be. Seizures were not really bad enough that he needed to go to the doctor or take medication, but Lola made him go to the doctor and take pills. Seizures were not dangerous enough that he should not drive, but Lola wouldn't let him drive. Seizures were not so severe that he could not do whatever he wanted, except Lola would not let him. Seizures were not the culprit behind the irrational behavior Lola says occurs, she just makes him mad. Therefore, the statement "I have never seen myself have a seizure" was not a bit funny to me. I knew exactly what it implied. Every time Charley stated those words I felt a sting in my heart and buried their implications beneath my sense of duty.

I took care of a man for more than twenty years who saw me as an imaginary enemy because he had never seen himself have a seizure. Charley lived with the bruises and bumps from falling and knew something was happening. He had no clue how out of control his body became when he had a seizure and did not know what role I played as his caretaker. The fact that I put aside my dreams to fulfill his, was sleep deprived and suffered many muscle strains from lifting or catching him during thousands of seizures never entered his mind.

I was the tattle-tale as far as Charley's irrational mind was concerned. There were times he implied if I had said nothing about seizures then they would not have existed. Deep down he knew better but his mind was flawed and lacked the ability to rationalize thoughts. I think everyone who is married to a person with a debilitating illness suffers greatly because there is no one else for the person who is ill to direct their disappointment and unhappiness toward.

However most illnesses can be seen and are acknowledged as real by the person who is sick. Not Charley. He had never seen himself have a seizure and the only person saying he had seizures ninety-nine percent of the time was Lola. In time Charley emanated an underlying resentment toward me. I lived his seizures and because of them forced Charley to tow the lines he always wanted to cross. Not a pretty picture for me any way you paint it but I stuck around because I committed to "in sickness and health" and I loved my husband dearly. Sometimes I considered videotaping Charley so he could see a seizure but never did because this was one more way I felt he needed protecting. The thought never occurred to me if Charley saw himself have a seizure he would also see me taking care of him.

The last time we traveled to Dallas when Charley was admitted to the Epilepsy Unit at Parkland I was fed up with the statement I see reality. Before we left the hospital I asked the staff if Charley could watch a video of himself having a seizure. I wanted him to see a seizure but did not think about him seeing what I did. I hoped he might realize the damage that something so severe could inflict after more than twenty years and understand his reality was flawed. I was willing to do anything to get past I see reality.

The nurses were very receptive to our watching the video and called us into a room where we could. Charley's attitude was poor as he smugly sat down to participate in one more thing I was forcing upon him. The film showed us both in the hospital room when he was monitored before surgery. Within a short time he had a seizure and as always we looked into each others' eyes and our souls began to communicate. His soul told mine his body was going out of control and my soul reassured his that I would keep him safe. During our entire marriage I had been the only person out of the two of us who had ever consciously experienced these moments of communication between our souls. Charley stared in silence as he watched his seizure and witnessed our spiritual communication. During this time his soul began reliving the same sense of panic he always involuntarily felt when seizures took over his body. Sitting in that room with me, though Charley was lucid, his soul called out to mine. My soul answered and I put my hand on his arm to calm him as I had always done. I placed my hand on his arm and at that moment he felt the reassurance he had always instinctively felt when a seizure was overtaking his body and his soul knew I was there to keep him safe. For the first time Charley saw the wordless communication between us and he could not deny the reassurance he felt as our spirits spoke.

Then Charley realized I was the main character in the film. He was on the bed having a seizure as I took care of him. He saw me wipe the slobber off his face, catch his urine, hold his hands, rub his arms, talk to him and ease him through the seizure. When the seizure was over he was sitting on the side of the bed and I was standing in front of him. As he had done thousands of times before Charley leaned his head against my tummy while I rubbed my fingers through his hair and spoke words of comfort.

Experiencing the communication between our souls deeply moved Charley. He was moved beyond the insanity we had taken him to Dallas for and beyond saying thank-you because he realized in his heart that would not begin to cover all my hardships. After twenty-four years of being blamed, misunderstood and unappreciated I was instantly no longer the imagined enemy. The entire tone of our relationship changed. Seeing a seizure and witnessing our silent communication helped Charley see reality and appreciate me.

Charley did not say a word for quite some time. He had tears in his eyes when he finally looked at me. Words were not necessary. My wounded soul quietly heard the words his anguished soul spoke. A few days after we returned home he thanked me from the bottom of his heart for taking care of him in spite of the fact that he had taken for granted the hardships his illness had placed upon me. I cried and cried and washed many years of pain out of my heart.

Watching that film did not completely put a halt to the phrase I see reality but it did help and brought Charley to a new level of understanding. He was more grateful. I can't advise anyone dealing with this same situation to film someone having a seizure and make them watch. The caretaker who is tuned into the person who has seizures can help with the decision of whether a person should actually see themselves have a seizure.

Charley was forced to acknowledge his seizures. That should have happened many years before. His mind was unable to accept his illness before he had surgery. After surgery he was a different person. It took baby steps to get him there but the new seizure-free world he lived in was much better than the old debilitating life he left behind. None of the events we experienced would have come about if he had not had brain surgery.

Charley viewing me as an imaginary enemy hurt my heart more than any other aspect of his illness. I buried the pain his unwarranted animosity caused for many years in order to take care of him. It hit the core of my being as I grieved the death of my husband when I realized that before brain surgery Charley unfairly perceived me as an imaginary enemy . . . and after surgery . . . he died before I could get accustomed to being his real friend.

Writing the Last Chapter Together

Chapter 26

Would I Do It Again?

When I tell people I am a widow they always ask what I am doing. Everyone knows the death of a spouse ends one life and begins another but I have yet to hear the unspoken words plainly stated. Three years have passed since Charley's death and my life has changed tremendously. I cannot let go of his spirit until this book is finished. Then I will spread his ashes high on top of our favorite mountain as I promised to him when he was dying so his spirit can be free.

When asked what I am doing I reveal that I am writing a book about how we lived with Charley's epilepsy. It is good to tell others about my project. When time goes by and I don't write I constantly remind myself to keep our memories alive until this book is completed. Though Charley is dead my heart is still very committed to him. When this book is finished I will heal from his life, and his death.

The thought of living with a person who had seizures and was psychotic puzzles people. I was married to a fascinating man whose progressive illness slowly robbed him of the life he deserved. Rather than lie down and die from seizures Charley chose to have the left temporal lobe of his brain removed with the dream of finally experiencing a normal life.

After briefly explaining his epilepsy and surgery many people have asked if I would do it again. Would I do it again? The question always leaves me perplexed. So many thoughts are stomping on each other as they run through my head that I cannot quickly formulate an honest answer.

When Charley was alive I pictured us sitting together finishing the last chapter of this book. I could hardly wait for his brain to heal and us to have lived a few years past the surgery. I anticipated asking him if he felt the surgery worth the sacrifices. Would he do it again? Would undergoing brain surgery to eliminate seizures be something Charley might encourage another person to do?

We are writing the last chapter together but in a different way than

I ever imagined. Shortly after Charley's death a dear friend of ours hand-made a wooden box to store Charley's ashes in. His initials, C.R.J. are embossed in varnished wood grain letters on the front of the box. A small black storage box slips into the top of the box that holds his ashes. Under the glass on the carved wooden lid of the small box is my favorite picture of Charley. Inside the smaller box is a note our granddaughter, Audrey, wrote to her Papa after he died and a cast iron turtle she wanted in the box with Papa's ashes to keep him company. Also in the small box are a few pictures of us laughing and having fun together. Right now that box containing Charley's ashes sits on the floor under my desk. Three years after beginning this book I sit alone, bare feet comfortably propped against my husband's box of ashes, while I write the final chapter of our journeys. The memories belonged to both of us. It is so hard to write the last chapter without Charley here to reminisce and laugh with but I will do my best to give him a voice.

I am sure Charley would say the surgery was worth the sacrifices. Life gave a lot back to him when he became seizure free and the most important things he did not even know were missing. His feelings, dreams and the ability to communicate on a subconscious level initially scared the hell out of him but he learned how to balance the new with the old and became a better man.

If we had been aware of how hard the adjustment to life without seizures was going to be for me I would have had counseling before the surgery. No one could have predicted the circumstances we underwent. Being prepared for the changes would have been an advantage but I do not believe anyone could have convinced me that my adjustments would be so difficult. We had to live and learn from those circumstances. Even considering those factors I believe Charley would have had the surgery. The insanity we endured after surgery was not anyone's fault any more than epilepsy or seizures were. Regardless of the negative factors I am glad Charley had brain surgery.

Charley and I speak together in saying to anyone who suffers with seizures not to take any seizure lightly. Don't take a chance and wait until so many years go by that you become psychotic and your mental capacity is forever damaged to find epilepsy specialists. We saw many physicians who prescribed medication for Charley with the hope of controlling his seizures. Not one of those doctors inquired about his psychosis even when we both tried to explain the insanity. They were not helpful with the negative behavioral aspects that can be a part of epilepsy.

The specialists at the epilepsy clinic at the University of Texas set a goal of eliminating Charley's seizures and met their goal. If we had gone to epilepsy specialists sooner perhaps Charley might have lived more seizure-free years and his psychosis may not have run rampant.

I am certain Charley would warn anyone considering brain surgery that the headaches after surgery were horrible. For a while he felt that he had traded seizures for headaches because he could not escape them. When he healed enough to get on an even keel the headaches stopped unless he became too tired. In time he learned a new system of pacing himself so he did not overexert his brain and cause a headache.

For some time I have been contemplating how to begin this chapter without Charley beside me. I read and corrected each chapter and asked myself over and over if I have fairly represented Charley and explained everything in a way that would be acceptable to him. The only information lacking is not accurately providing what Charley was feeling from the inside out as he lived with epilepsy. How could I?

Last week a sudden unexplainable urge to clean out a shed that has not been cleaned since before Charley died consumed me. I think a soul was quietly whispering to mine once again. After several hours of ignoring the urge I found myself in that building sorting through and throwing away piles of junk. Then I found a dusty box of paperwork that contained medical records from the 1990's. Within this box I spied several pieces of paper with Charley's handwriting on them. I turned a bucket upside down and sat on it. In that dust-filled shed with tears making tracks down my dirty face I slowly read what Charley had written. Notes from a ghost, placed in my hands by his spirit, irreplaceable words written by my husband nineteen years ago. Charley was well enough then to comprehend his illness. Our life did not start out with him incapacitated. That happened gradually over the years.

Charley always got a kick out of interrupting me when I was babbling and telling me to be quiet because it was his turn to talk. I believe his soul was telling mine that once again. I will be quiet one last time and let my Charley talk.

1-12-91

O'boy. Another one of these nights. I'm going to try my best to be understandable with this to the point of being so understandable that hopefully someone who doesn't even know what epilepsy is can understand and know what I feel like is going on in my head. One must constantly bear in mind that my literary talent is that of a carpenter.

My first experience is that of waking up in the hospital wondering where I was, and just what was going on. I couldn't move. Everything started going pretty fast then. Why couldn't I move and where in the hell could I be? I was in a straight-jacket. My beautiful wife, who has stuck by me through this all, started explaining to me that I had a seizure (whatever that was) and she had called an ambulance and they had taken me here to the hospital. Apparently, because of my lack of this kind of experience before, they had no idea of what was going on either and had me restrained with the straight-jacket. After much screaming and verbal violence they decided that I was coherent and the Dr. on duty had OK'ed my release from the restraints (Thank God). After a minor verbal inquiry I was released from the hospital. Boy, did I feel like I had suffered a drunken beating. Confused, but feeling much better within the week I saw another doctor and was Rx'd Dilantin and Valproic Acid (approx 600 mg. each). I really felt like my crazy young adulthood was screaming at me.

Needless to say, I experienced the seizure again. I always seemed to have them in my sleep. They seemed to occur about once a month. The headaches and neck cramps were tremendous afterwards. Soon the headaches were coming before the seizures. Before long I could almost tell when I was going to have one.

Having no personal physician other than the family physician I eventually went to him. He being a D.O. doctor.

I soon discovered that being a vet did have its advantages and got into the V.A. Hospital for a diagnosis. After seeing as many as a dozen Dr's over the next 18 months was released from the V.A. Hospital.

Back to the grind of hustling medical help for myself. By now 18 or 19 months had passed and I was finally diagnosed as having epilepsy. What a relief to finally know what the monster that had me was named. Although at this point I'm not so sure that this diagnoses was going to be easy to deal with (it never has been).

The seizures have always given me a premonition of their arrival. I've always gotten signals that they were trying to happen. Although, most have been in my sleep. The attempts of a seizure to overcome me feels like basically the same thing. It is difficult to explain, especially to someone who has never suffered one. It seems to feel like a blankness trying to overcome me. Like the darkness overcoming the earth at dusk. Fighting it back sometimes takes all the mental power of my consciousness to do. This is a mostly unconscious effort. It leaves me with a severe neck cramp in the back and base of my neck. Sometimes before and after a seizure an intense headache through the temples along with the neck cramp persists. Through the 10 – 11 years that I suffered this phenomenon I have averaged a seizure approximately one every 3 – 5 weeks. Sometimes have gone as long as 6 months without one or as many as 6 – 7 in one day.

As I learn more about this monster I can still only describe the sensation in a poor way. I don't know if it's due to my lack of descriptive adjectives or the actual affliction keeping me so distant from the descriptive words. The affliction seems to have grown in as much as I now have moments when I stare off in space and have lost all memory and concept of time.

The sensation of a seizure is that of helplessness and fear. Basically all the seizures that I've had where I go out feel all the same. They apparently originate from the same place and it feels as if that place is growing. I have experienced not being able to talk. This feels really weird. It is formulated correctly in the brain but gets jumbled before it comes out of my mouth. After repeating it several times, it still comes out my mouth as jumble. I have spoken sentences in which I have said a jumbled word instead of the correct one. Also jumbled on a repeat of the sentence. Sometimes I hear words incorrectly as well as say words incorrectly. Apparently I hear others speaking in the wrong tone of voice as well because I sometimes get angry at, not necessarily what is said, but the manner in which it's said. I attribute a lot of this to the way I feel about having this affliction. I really miss being the ol' happy-go-lucky I used to be. When I get tired, the eyes are really hard to focus on exactly what I'm looking at, although I can see it seeing the whole room. This is the same way I operate more and more often now. I seem to see the whole room instead of what I'm exactly looking at; somewhat of a fixed stare. It's almost the same sensation as experiencing an out out-of -body sensation. Like looking at every one in the room, including myself, from the position of hanging from the light fixture. This I describe as Petit Mal. An Aura I describe as seeing something that has multi-outlines like rings in water that has something dropped in it. Sometimes I have experienced both of these at the same time.

1-14-91

Good morning. I seizured last night. The headache is tremendous this morning although the sensations of life are more distinct this morning. Water, coffee, roll and everything are very distinctive tasting and separate tasting. Normally the taste of things is combined to maybe one taste. This is normal. At the present things are independently and distinctive tasting. This is an unusually funny sensation. My vocabulary doesn't seem to want to flow. The headache through the temples is tremendous.

God, please join my side today. I love life and don't want to lose it. I am physically exhausted and tired. I don't seem to have any energy.

Charley Jines – 1991

Darkness overcoming the earth at dusk within your head, fighting seizures with all of your mental power, severe neck cramps, intense headaches, living with a monster ruling your life, lost memory and concept of time, constant feelings of helplessness and fear, the inability to speak, misunderstood anger, fixed stares, out of body sensations, total exhaustion and the constant fear of losing your life. That is only a small part of what epilepsy forced Charley to endure.

No one deserves to fight such battles every day. I thank Dr. Diaz Arrastia and Dr. Mickey and all the staff at the University of Texas. You, and the two years of seizure-free life you gave Charley, were truly a gift from God.

Dear Charley,

I don't cry as often but I do cry at times because I miss you. I am sorry you lost your life but I know your prayers are answered. God joined your side forever, you are whole again and your suffering is over. Now that I have finished writing our story I am going to spread your ashes on top of our favorite mountain and let your spirit go. Our memories I will cherish forever. Your soul will quietly speak to mine from time to time and mine will answer, as it always has.

I pray it brings you peace and comfort when you hear my spirit say,

"My Charley,
I will always adore you.
Yes, I would do it again.